THE MENOPAUSE PLAN

Dear Violet
Best Wishes
3-15-17

THE MENOPAUSE PLAN

A GUIDE TO AGING GRACEFULLY AND MAINTAINING SEXUAL VIBRANCY

Dr. Tracey Jayne Fein M.D.
Board Certified Obstetrician-Gynecologist
Senior Attending Physician,
Lenox Hill Hospital, N.Y.C.
25 years in clinical practice.

TheMenopausePlan.com

Medical Disclaimer
The information presented in this book is the result is the result of years of clinical practice experi-
ence by the author. The information in this book, by necessity, is of a general nature and not a
substitute for an evaluation, examination or treatment by a competent medical specialist. If you
believe you are in need of medical treatment please see a medical practitioner as soon as possible.
The stories in this book are true. The names and circumstances of the stories have been changed
to protect the anonymity of patients.

Cover designed by Stefan Killen 3 Jay Street Brooklyn NY
Stefankillen.com

The Library of Congress has cataloged this edition as follows:
Fein, Tracey
The Menopause Plan/Dr. Tracey Fein M.D.
ISBN-13: 9780997803402 (custom)
ISBN-10: 0997803401
1. Educational   2. Self-Help   3. Women's Studies   4. Medical

Books may be purchased for educational, business or promotional use. For information on bulk
purchases, please contact sales at drtraceyfein@gmail.com
First published in the United States by Osprey Hill Press.
First edition 2016.

A DOCTOR'S NOTE

PRACTICING MEDICINE IN New York City over the past twenty-five years has allowed me to meet and help thousands of women as they experienced menopause. Every woman I treated was unique and had specific likes, dislikes and preferences for treatment. Treating women individually is the heart of The Menopause Plan as every woman experiences the effects of menopause differently.

Frequently, the most important time spent between myself and a patient is speaking about what is happening with their bodies and what the future holds for them going forward. The women you are about to meet in The Menopause Plan range in age from forty-three years old to seventy-nine years of age. Each one experienced menopause in a unique way because each experience of menopause is unique. Their stories help illuminate the great variety of ways that menopause effects women and outlines the most effective treatments at each stage of menopause.

My own story of menopause serves as a prime example of a fifty-five year old woman who delayed early treatment and suffered adverse effects. With proper treatment the worst effects of my menopause were reversed and the story of my own journey into menopause had a very positive outcome after a very dramatic beginning.

CHAPTER 1

MENOPAUSE NEEDS A plan. A scientifically valid, medically beneficial, proven effective, safe plan to help guide women from forty years of age into their senior years. During this time a woman's body undergoes significant physical changes as estrogen levels begin to diminish before eventually ceasing production altogether. Left untreated falling estrogen levels result in a progressive loss of sexual function, reduced ability to achieve orgasms and vaginal atrophy leading to dry, thin tissues that become prone to bladder and vaginal infections. This is true for all women.

Therefore treating menopause means preventing vaginal atrophy. Treatment should begin as early as possible and continue into the senior years for as long as practical because left untreated, the progression of vaginal atrophy due to the absence of estrogen has no end date.

The experience of sex and of being a sexual person exists as a kind of flow state that accompanies us as we make our way through life. Not one of us carries an expectation that there will come a day when our sex lives have ended and yet for many women this is in fact what happens. The gradual erosion of sexuality and sexual health is the end result of undiagnosed, untreated or inadequately treated symptoms of estrogen depletion as a result of menopause.

By understanding menopause's deep complexities we can create a grand strategy helping us age gracefully while keeping our sexual vibrancy through this period of naturally occurring hormonal imbalances. Generating a plan for future good health is dependent on understanding both the timeframe and scope these changes occur within.

Most people have a strategy for maintaining good heart health; they avoid certain foods, perhaps they exercise or take medications if lab results so indicate. Good dental health is also something we form a program to achieve by brushing, flossing and having regular checkups that begin at an early age. On the matter of good vaginal health however, there has been no central guiding principle or established plan for fighting vaginal atrophy. This particular symptom is perhaps both the most destructive aspect of menopause and the least understood.

Physicians whose patients are undergoing menopause frequently offer treatments for symptoms such as skipped periods, hot flashes, sleeplessness, loss of libido and so forth. Medications, herbal treatments and creams of various types are prescribed to alleviate these uncomfortable, yet transitory effects of the change of life. In other words, both doctors and patients typically chase symptoms seeking relief as each symptom appears. Menopause is often regarded as a constellation of transitory symptoms requiring temporary medications for relief, while the permanent damage that occurs due to the lack of estrogen is ignored.

Without estrogen, the cells making up the walls of the vagina change. As vaginal tissues age they will no longer be replaced by new tissue growth as happens in younger women who are still producing abundant estrogen. The cellular growth that creates healthy vaginal tissue requires estrogen, without it the walls of the vagina gradually become thin, sex becomes difficult, painful and eventually impossible.

As the pleasure of sex fades the desire for it also fades. By the senior years, a vagina that has been untreated becomes dysfunctional, very dry, with skin that is prone to irritation and infections. Therefore, treating menopause effectively means preventing vaginal atrophy before bad things happen and sexual dysfunction becomes established. Prevention is as always, the best cure.

KATHERINE

Katherine is 52 years old with a very classic New York put-together look about her. It had been a few years since she'd seen an ob-gyn and it was the first time I'd met her. Before the examination, blood tests and routine stuff began, we sat and talked for a little while.

"Hi thanks for coming its nice to meet you," I said extending my hand, "What brings you in today?"

"Hello Dr. Fein. I figure its time for a checkup."

"First, how are you feeling? Are there any urgent medical issues or health problems you'd like to talk about?"

"No not really, I feel fine."

"Good, so tell me a little about yourself."

"I'm in banking and I work for JP Morgan Chase down at Wall Street. I've got a Yorkshire terrier named Smitty. Divorced, two kids. I do photography, Yoga.

"How old are the kids?" I asked.

Katherine pulled out her phone and showed me the screen, "Mickey's ten and Marisa's just turned fourteen."

"Disneyland?" I asked pointing to the background.

"Yup, Mickey wanted to meet his namesake."

"You named him after Mickey Mouse?" I asked.

"No, we named him after his Uncle Mickey but he thinks he was named after Mickey Mouse so we're leaving it at that for the time being."

"If I was ten that's how I'd roll."

"Exactly," Katherine said.

"So," I said picking up Katherine's folder, "It sounds like you're here for a routine exam and checkup, do you have any medical or gynecological history I should know about? Ever been in the hospital for anything? Sickness, operation or accident?"

"No, no and no."

"Any problems going to the bathroom, urinating or moving your bowels?" She nodded no, "Do you take medications or have a history of any bad reaction or allergy to a drug or medicine?"

"No not at all."

"What about your period?"

"Stopped about five years ago."

"Did you receive any treatments, medications or hormone replacements?" I asked.

"No again."

"Are you in a relationship and are you sexually active?" I asked.

"Actually," Katherine said taking a moment to get started, "That's where it gets a little complicated. I got divorced about five years ago and didn't really want to meet anyone let alone do the whole dating thing," She hesitated then continued making eye contact, "But that changed and I met a guy online and I've been seeing him for a few weeks. We get along really great, I like him, and he's super nice…"

"And?" I asked.

"Last week we went to bed and it was a total disaster. I mean it hurt. I was like 'Stop, we have to stop' and he was so apologetic and concerned that he hurt me. I got so upset I cried and ohmigosh, talk about a way to lose a guy in two minutes flat and that's got to be at the top. I mean the first time I'm having sex in five years and it goes like this? What the hell?"

I swear I wanted to hug her. We spoke for a few minutes more and then went to the exam room for a quick look and some tests but I already had a good idea what was going on. By age 52 unless a woman has been treated for estrogen depletion, her vagina will already be in trouble.

"See anything down there?" Katherine asked, her feet up in stirrups.

I gestured that she could put her feet down and get dressed, "Yes, you have menopause and its time for us to make a plan about how to treat it."

"Did you see any reason why intercourse hurt?"

"Oh yes," I said, "I did indeed."

And from that jumping off point Katherine and I started a discussion that ranged from hot flashes (She didn't have them) to skipped periods (Hers just stopped) insomnia (Never) and irritability (Always, but not likely related to menopause, she said).

"Kids?" I asked.

"Bingo!" She replied, "So tell me, why exactly was sex so painful?" Katherine asked.

I sat back in my chair and took a breath, "The complicated answer is that estrogen diminishes after menopause. Without estrogen vaginal tissue becomes dry and thin, left untreated this condition makes intercourse painful, difficult and eventually impossible. The condition is called vaginal atrophy." I paused for a moment because Katherine's expression became markedly distressed. "It happens to all women during and after menopause and it's progressive. It gets a little worse each year. The good news is, its very treatable especially in the early stage you're at now." Katherine looked up at me.

"It's progressive?" She asked.

"That's why it's important to get treated, the earlier the better. It's very likely that if we'd started medication a few years ago you might not have had problems with sex at all. Preventing those kinds of things in the future is what we'll try and achieve with your Menopause Plan. But for starters, let's try a low dosage vaginal estrogen cream it needs to be applied three times a week after an initial two weeks of daily usage. This will lessen the symptoms and make you feel much better. How much better we can only say after its had time to work. The result should be improved vaginal tissue health and easier sex. Give it about a month and then I'll predict you won't have another bad sex episode."

Katherine looked at me with uncertainty and I said, "It'll be ok, it really will. We can treat this. You can have great sex after menopause. Really." I said.

Katherine's experience of menopause was unique to her. The common symptoms that most women suffer were not present in her case. There was no need for herbal remedies to help with hot flashes, pills for insomnia, meditation techniques or SSRI's for dealing with emotional issues. Her experience of menopause included a lover and the desire to express physical intimacy.

For Katherine the largest negative effect of menopause was that her ability to have a physical relationship was compromised due to unexpected medical issues. As a doctor and as a woman it is difficult to witness the complexities of human life as things like this unfold. Pain of course can be physical but it can be emotional too and that is what I saw when I treated Katherine. Her physical symptoms caused real pain but the greater pain was the heartache that the painful sex caused.

There is an undeniable connection between mind and body. If life becomes difficult for the body the mind will also suffer. This is why a Menopause Plan becomes an effective tool for reducing suffering of both the mind and the body. It enables women to make a plan to avoid future suffering.

Preventing menopause from becoming a negative experience marked by loss, difficult sex and stressed relationships should be our collective goal as patients and doctors. By preventing these effects of menopause from taking hold, later heartache can be avoided. And this is the skill of a good life, avoiding things that will cause bad results. In Katherine's case the thing she might have done to avoid later problems was to seek early treatment for vaginal atrophy. She did not know that she had it, it came to her silently and only announced itself when sex had become painful causing her tears that she need not have shed.

The Doctor's Best Advice that I can offer is to get checked early, get treated appropriately and make a plan. Menopause specialists can prevent sexual health from declining and can reverse its worst effects through medications and other treatments such as laser rejuvenation. It is possible after menopause to regrow soft, moist vaginal tissue like that found in younger women and it's also possible to have great sex after menopause. But it cannot happen on it's own. For that you need a doctor and a plan.

The Silent Menace of Menopause

The constellation of symptoms that women usually identify as "Menopause" masks the fundamental truth of what is really going on in a woman's body. The silent menace of menopause is vaginal atrophy resulting in sexual dysfunction that may begin as early as forty years old and continues unabated into the senior years. After menopause begins, these tissues begin to change making sex painful, difficult or impossible. These changes are subtle and take place gradually over a long period of time, making them hard to see for what they are.

As a result women frequently attribute the symptoms of vaginal atrophy to yeast infections, loss of libido or temporary dryness. As sexual dysfunction becomes more established, a woman's desire fades as sex is no longer pleasurable and orgasms become difficult to achieve. This is the reality of menopause.

Left untreated all women will eventually become sexually dysfunctional and increasingly prone to infection. Vaginal deterioration is inevitable; it is progressive and starts with the onset of menopause. By the time a woman has hot flashes she already has vaginal atrophy.

Chasing after symptoms like hot flashes does nothing to prevent the degradation of vaginal health. The outward, troubling effects of menopause like sleeplessness etc., can be treated effectively with a wide range of beneficial medications. However, while those symptoms may improve, lessen or go away, vaginal atrophy continues year after year eventually resulting in the loss of sexual function. In the senior years vaginal tissue becomes increasingly dry, thin and prone to bladder and vaginal infections that can have a major impact on overall health and quality of life.

Treating menopause therefore means keeping and maintaining vaginal health as a priority as a woman experiences the decades long process of menopause. There are many safe, effective treatments with different approaches being best at different times. That is why every woman needs a Menopause Plan. Managing menopause effectively, especially vaginal health, is the key to aging gracefully and maintaining sexual vibrancy.

SOFIA

Sofia was 43 years old when we first met about five years ago. A graduate of Parsons School of Design and a fashion consultant by trade, she was the type of chic New York lady you see on the street and think, "Is that someone famous?" Sofia just had that aura about her.

New patients on their first visit need a little more time for us to get to know one another. After some small talk I began to ask about her family background, sexual history and health issues that already exist, then we moved on to the physical exam.

Sofia got dressed after the exam and we teamed up back in my office where we started to talk about some of the things that came up earlier.

She sat opposite me in the armchair and in reply to my inquiry about her periods she said, "I started skipping them about six months ago but I just chalked it up to the usual stress, emotional overload kind of thing. I wasn't in a relationship so possibly being pregnant wasn't relevant."

"Didn't you say you were getting hot flashes too?" I asked.

"Umm hmmm."

"So you know pre-menopause has started right?" I said making a note in the file.

"Menopause started," Sofia said in a flat voice, "At forty-three?"

"At forty-three. As early as the late thirties in some women but the more common age is around fifty. You're one of the early starters and it'd be best if we came up with a way to guide you through the coming years ahead. Because once it starts, you know, it just keeps marching along."

"I'm a vegan. I'm a fitness buff. I watch every thing I eat. Everything as organic and natural as possible."

"All good things," I said "But they can't reverse or stop the effects of menopause."

"I mean it more in the sense of that I don't want to take hormones."

"I understand and yet the source of the hot flashes, early onset of menopause and eventually vaginal dryness, sex problems and so on is that there is not enough estrogen in your body to keep you healthy."

"I'm frankly worried about taking something that could hurt me in the future," Sofia explained.

"Ok, I completely understand your preferences. But just hear me out for a second. Low dose estrogen is perfectly safe and will keep you in good health while your body goes though these changes. Without estrogen the hormonal balance of a woman's body is knocked out of whack. Sometimes women hear about treatments like this and they become concerned because there was once an over-prescription of these medications where they were used as a generalized cure-all for women going through menopause." Sofia nodded her head to acknowledge that she knew these things.

"That's not what we're talking about here," I continued, "This is a precise application of a safe effective treatment for the express purpose of hormonal rebalancing. As your natural ability to produce these chemicals diminishes bad things start to happen to your vagina and sex drive. The treatment I think will work best for you will prevent vaginal atrophy and keep you in good health for decades to come."

"Dr. Fein I really appreciate that," Sofia began, "But here's the thing, first I'm going to be happy when my periods stop. I hated them from the first one I ever got, so like goodbye and good riddance. And two, the hot flashes are only an annoyance. I don't get stopped dead in my tracks, I'm not tearing off my clothes, I'm not waking up in the middle of the night in January and turning on the air-conditioning. They suck but so do a lot of things and that's the category I'm putting them in, 'Tolerable things that suck'. To which I'll also add that eventual vaginal whatever is less scary to me than taking hormones now. Here's my viewpoint, I understand about estrogen but from my research I find it unappealing, it's too Big Pharma, it's a chemical. I'm trying to keep everything natural that I put in my body."

I thought she put it very well. Sofia certainly doesn't need me to tell her how to live her life, I'm only here to help in whatever way may be beneficial. And so despite my reservations, I knew it was time to move on, but first I said, "Totally ok with me. The only take-away I want to leave you with is that menopause ends with vaginal atrophy and sexual dysfunction, it happens in all women. Early treatment is the best treatment. And that's it end of lecture. Now let me ask you," I said changing the subject to another important topic, "You said your Mom has Type 2 diabetes do I remember right?"

"Yes she does."

"Do you need to urinate frequently?" I asked.

"No."

"Good. We'll do a Hemoglobin A1C blood test that will show us if your average blood sugar over the last three months has been elevated. It's a good precaution given your family history. The reason for the question about increased urination is because diabetics sometimes have that symptom but it's also a common symptom of a urinary tract infection."

"God I hope I don't have diabetes," Sofia said before adding, "Or a urinary tract infection for that matter. Either."

"Your health habits are good and from what you've told me and what I've observed I think you're ok. The test is only a precautionary thing because you don't want an imbalance in your body chemistry wreaking havoc with your internal parts like diabetes."

"Don't say it 'Or like estrogen for your vagina'."

"I wasn't going to say it," I said. We talked a little more, I gave her a prescription for an ongoing minor issue and she put her coat on, said goodbye, waved and left. The truth was that I was totally going to say that insulin is a hormone and when you have an imbalance like with diabetes it causes problems, just like happens to a vagina undergoing estrogen depletion. But, she beat me to it and I had to retreat.

Sofia has strong opinions that help her formulate ideas about her health and health needs. Some of these ideas are sound, like her choices for a vegan diet and regular exercise and others are ideas she picked up from her own research, a magazine article, TV or the internet. Her aversion to estrogen is not uncommon among women I see who have received news about health topics based on incomplete analyses or just sometimes, incorrect reporting.

Sifting through all the medical news, data, science, lab results, individual variations and figuring out what works best for whom and in what circumstance is the work of a physician menopause specialist. Offering Sofia a low dose of estrogen treatment was not what she wanted, it did not fit into her overall way of thinking about natural and organic ways to live and maintain health. I respect that and I respect her.

But there is a larger truth that is evident to a physician meno-pause specialist who has treated thousands of women over decades of time, when a woman starts menopause early her symptoms later on will be more severe. I have seen many cases just like Sofia's where the offer of treatment was declined. My assertive nature in trying to have Sofia reach acceptance of this treatment was due to the fact that I know what happens to a vagina when it no longer has access to estro-gen. Eventually sexual and relationship issues emerge. Infections become more common. These effects can be minimized by early intervention.

Unfortunately the cumulative effects of estrogen depletion cannot be alleviated by healthy diets or frequent exercise alone but estrogen or hormone balancing treatments in women experiencing early pre-meno-pause can be safe and highly effective in reducing symptoms short term and delaying or preventing unwanted sexual problems.

SEX

<u>Viagra for him. Headaches for her.</u>

Sex is the one of the great motivators of human beings. It exists on the level of physical attraction, orgasms and reproduction but also exists on the level of basic biology. Nowhere is this more apparent than in the current imbalance between medications such as Viagra for men and the lack of an equivalent treatment for women. In spite of recent media hype, there is no female Viagra and there may never be because the inherent qualities that lead to sexual arousal in women are far more complicated than those present in men.

This is a classic example of the Battle of the Sexes fought out in the bedroom. Men have their sexual needs and specific medications to

help those needs are widely available. Men who have difficulty becoming sexually aroused can take a pill and attain an erection. Women
have no such recourse. There is no vaginal version of an erection pill
and the thought of a partner with outsized sexual needs forces many
women to contemplate the inherent unfairness of life. So let's take a
look at sexual arousal and the different processes between men and
women.

For men it's all about erections; getting them and keeping them
long enough to reach orgasm. Treating erectile dysfunction, as a man
gets older is a positive step in maintaining sexual vitality and a positive
self-image. Expressing love through physical intimacy is something that
brings joy to couples and helps to bind them together more tightly. More
erections on a regular and sustainable basis should therefore be a positive step toward better sex and a more lasting union. Right?

Well, only sometimes. You see here's the issue. Many men begin to
lose sexual vibrancy as they get into their forties, fifties and beyond.
They may retain the desire for sexual relations, but the ability to have
and or maintain erections begins to dwindle due to conditions that
restrict blood flow. Men have a sexual response cycle that is far more
simple and direct than do women. As men get sexually aroused, blood
begins to flow to their private parts and an erection occurs. They are
ready for sexual intercourse. This is the mechanism that all the erectile
dysfunction drugs address, how to increase blood flow to the penis.

Women have another whole thing going on as the loss of estrogen
provokes an entire range of sexual maladies. With reduced new vaginal
tissue growth, the results are dryness, painful sex, discomfort, loss of
libido and a reduced ability to experience sexual pleasure. There is no
pill that quickly increases women's sexual desire and functioning the
way Viagra fixes erectile dysfunction. For a woman to be fully sexual, her
vagina needs the types of cell growth that creates elastic, strong vaginal
tissue capable of experiencing sexual feelings.

And there lies the problem. Viagra for him and vaginal dryness accompanied by painful sex for her. We need to admit there is a

mismatch in pharmaceutical heaven somewhere. The men are ready and the women could use a little help.

But there is no real Viagra for women and the reason lies in the complicated nature of women's sexuality compared to men's sexuality. To feel sexy a man needs an erection that he can get by popping a pill. To feel equally sexy a woman needs a vagina that creates pleasurable sensations during sex.

Vaginal Atrophy vs. Four-Hour Erections? Please. You'll be the one seeking medical attention, forget about him.

For women who wish to retain sexual vibrancy through menopause without hormones there is a new, safe treatment that has proven highly effective. The procedure utilizes a medical laser similar to what plastic surgeons use for facial rejuvenation for eliminating laugh lines and wrinkles. When used on vaginal tissue, the laser zaps the older tissue exciting it to regrow with softer, moister more abundant skin cells with better blood supply like those found in younger women who are still producing estrogen.

This recent development in treating menopausal symptoms is generating buzz because it is the first effective treatment resulting in better sexual function and greater sexual desire. Desire for sex is seen to increase in relation to the frequency that a woman experiences pleasurable sex. The better the sexual experience, the more one will wish to experience it again.

Viagra for him. Vaginal rejuvenation for her. The best news to come from the frontiers of medicine regarding women's sexuality is that there is now a way to achieve equality between the male oriented drugs that increase sexual vibrancy in men and the vaginal rejuvenation treatments that increase sexual vibrancy in women. In the war of the sexes, this should be heralded as one of the more successful outcomes in the struggle for equality from the bedroom to the boardroom.

ORGASMS

Sex is about a lot of things. Love, intimacy, physical pleasure and of course, the final topping on the sundae of a good relationship has to be good orgasms.

For women, they are widely reported to come in two flavors, clitoral and vaginal and so its natural to ask why if vaginal atrophy eliminates one pathway to orgasm why does that matter if the clitoral pathway remains open? The answer is layered and complex because women's sexuality is layered and complex. With men the sex response is direct. With women it begins with hormones that trigger sexual feelings in the brain that also sends sexually responsive signals to their private parts. Women need both their brains and their vaginas to be stimulated for sex to be most pleasurable. For both sexy mental and physical stimulation to occur, the right balance of hormones and responsive tissue needs to be present. If they're absent sex simply won't be desired, fun or even in some cases, possible.

But that doesn't address the question of clitoral stimulation being a second pathway to orgasm mitigating the need for treating vaginal atrophy.

The answer is that orgasms for many women are the result of multiple areas of simultaneous stimulation and to remove one of the centers that provides sexual pleasure reduces or eliminates the possibility of satisfying orgasms. For many women if you take away vaginal stimulation the orgasmic response becomes more difficult to achieve.

MADELINE

Madeline's husband runs a hedge fund and her life's work revolves around family and philanthropic work. Originally from California she's been making New York her home since she got married right after college. She's 47 years old now and she's been my patient since she was 38, together we've worked our way through a variety of illnesses and conditions over the years.

Like half of all women over 40, Madeline developed fibroids in her uterus and they gave her increasing trouble as the years passed. Fibroids are benign tumors that grow within the uterus and they're very common. They are usually multiple and sometimes they can be large but cause few problems and sometimes they're small and cause real problems like pain and heavy bleeding depending on their location. They typically grow slowly and steadily until menopause.

In Madeline's case there was no need for surgery to remove them. They weren't in the way of anything vital and she experienced no pain. The best strategy was to deal with the symptoms she had, which was heavy bleeding and then wait for menopause to reduce her estrogen levels. As hormonal levels drop in menopause, for most women bleeding from fibroids will get better on its own. Madeline, we'd expect should be happier than most women to begin menopause because it meant that the fibroid problem would start to resolve.

But a complication arose. As Madeline's estrogen levels dropped, she became increasingly unhappy. Her state of mind became anxious and tense she became self-aware that her mental afflictions were without apparent causality. She was having an emotional reaction in her brain as her hormone levels became erratic as a result of pre-menopause.

We know that the mind-body connection is so strong that the slightest changes in hormones, physical environment, stress or sleep patterns can disrupt normal functioning. Sometimes this is a temporary condition that rights itself over time and in other cases the changes do not get better unless treated.

With Madeline we had a quandary on our hands. Her mental state was being afflicted by the changes of menopause and she could not take estrogen without risking developing more serious problems with fibroids that might result in a surgical solution becoming inevitable. Avoiding surgery is of course in everyone's best interest. Yet feeling anxious and

confused without being able to stop these unwanted feelings from arising can make a woman feel like she's going a little crazy. And avoiding
mental distress is also in everyone's best interest.

It was somewhat ironic, because for Madeline some aspects of the
onset of menopause were fine with her. She said she wouldn't miss having her periods and she also knew that the many years she had been
dealing with bleeding fibroids would get better. What arose was unexpected and the quandary we needed to find a way out of was that fibroids
feed on estrogen and usually diminish by themselves in its absence. As
Madeline began to run out of estrogen her brain chemistry changed
leading to afflictive states of mind. Adding estrogen to her body would
have alleviated the symptoms but was not a good option, as it could
make the fibroids worse.

Menopause, as we can see is complex. The effects on a woman's
body are highly individualistic and so therefore the treatments that are
used must be uniquely crafted for each woman. As a patient I'd known
for many years, the changes to Madeline's demeanor and the way she
answered my questions in a yearly examination made me immediately
concerned and we talked for a while about the best way to treat her
condition.

We looked at one another over my desk and Madeline's face was
more worried than I'd ever seen before, "When did it start?" I asked.

"It was right after Christmas," Madeline said as she fingered the top
button of her blouse, "I woke up in the middle of the night with this feeling that something was terribly wrong. Almost like a panic attack, it was
like a very strong emotion, like total stress just crashing over me like a
wave. I felt unfocused, hard to concentrate, worried. Anxious. So I got
up. Walked around. Waited half an hour. Drank a glass of wine and it
just went on and on. It would stop then kick back up again".

"How long did it last for?"

"Honestly?" Madeline said looking right at me, "It never went away
completely. I feel a little background buzz of it right now. Sometimes it
flares up, calms down, flares up, goes nuclear. Stops. Starts up again

six hours later or comes on me at two a.m., at this point I'm totally con-fused. I don't know why it comes and I don't know why it goes," She said. "So, Dr. Fein what's going on with me? Am I going crazy?"

If I didn't know Madeline very well and hadn't been treating her for so many years, I might have thought about tests to see if in fact her mental stability was in question. But I didn't have any genuine concern in this regard. Her mental state fit perfectly with the time of life she was in, her underlying condition and she had numerous factors that were most likely the cause of her worries. Certainly if I had detected anything else I would have pursued it, but my experience of being her longtime physician led my thoughts into another direction.

"No I don't think you're going crazy," I said. "But it might feel a little like you're losing control. Let's consider this an important thing to deal with but not the type of thing that's going to require a straitjacket. What I see happening is that your train of thought has started to switch tracks uncontrollably creating both anxiety and confusion. The inability to focus or stay on task you mentioned earlier is also something that makes people feel like they're becoming unhinged but here's what's really going on. A woman's mind and her body are deeply linked together, bound by cycles of hormones that come and go sometimes on a daily basis and some over decades. The effects on a woman's body vary widely and the cause and effect nature of symptoms, their causes and cures can be elusive. Fortunately, we know how to deal with this and here's what we can do starting today."

Madeline and I made eye contact "First, tell me about your fitness routine, do you go to the gym, do yoga?" I asked.

"Not really my thing," She said.

"It's best if it becomes something you make time for in your life," I replied, "The first prescription I'm writing for you is to become active because exercise will help rebalance your emotions and how you respond to your changing hormone levels. Studies have shown this is effective but is also a short-term benefit. To feel better you will need to do Yoga or some other activity everyday and the task of finding what kind of activity is acceptable for you is the task ahead. The second prescription is for MBSR,"

"Which is what?"

"Mindfulness Based Stress Reduction. It's a way to calm stressful conditions with the power of your mind. It's been proven that by concentrating your mind correctly a person can change the way their brain produces the chemicals effecting mood. In other words, by channeling your thoughts properly it is possible to change the way your body works, it's possible to move the mind away from afflictive states and into more wholesome states.

These two approaches, daily exercise and MBSR will help you as much as many medicines. At the same time we'll also start you on a calming herbal supplement that should reduce the symptoms of anxiety and confusion we were talking about."

"Not exactly what I was expecting."

"What were you expecting?"

"Prozac, Valium and maybe a handout on the benefits of electro-shock therapy." Madeline said.

"Let's not go there," I said writing down some referrals for a woman menopause Yoga expert and another for an MBSR specialist. "If these don't work we can talk about a prescription for a low dose SSRI medicine. Come back and see me in about a month. Call me immediately if anything changes or you find stuff too hard to deal with, don't go into crisis and suffer until you see me again cause you think I'll be annoyed. I won't. Call me. Promise?"

She nodded her head yes and as I came around the desk she wrapped me in her arms and gave me a big hug. It was the nicest thing that happened to me all day.

Complex & Hard to Figure Out

Even if you could solve Rubik's Cube in one minute flat you still wouldn't be able to unlock the mysteries of estrogen and the complexities of its interactions within a woman's body. Albert Einstein himself would emerge from a gynecology lecture on the subject shaking his head and thanking his lucky stars he only had to grapple with Relativity and spacetime.

What we know is that estrogen doesn't just play a role in the cycles of reproduction and menopause it plays a role in well, maybe everything. There are at least eight different important hormones that are affected by the rise or fall of estrogen in the blood stream, cellular structures and the brain. Most women become accustomed to dealing with cyclic and predictable hormone changes over time. What happens with pre-menopause is that hormonal fluctuations can be more extreme and less predictable creating an unwanted series of symptoms.

The complicated nature of coming up with a Menopause Plan is these many different chemicals interact with one another causing them in turn to change other hormonal balances. This creates a cascade of events that is difficult to unravel. Due to the multiplying effect of inter-related chemical responses it's just plain difficult to say that this symptom is the absolute effect of that cause.

A certain symptom may be attributable to a single hormone, two hormones interacting, or many of them acting together. They can be at different levels of strength in relation to one another or they can vary all by themselves; and of course they can change due to natural variations throughout the day such as circadian rhythms and other forces over longer periods of time. The same hormone changes will also likely produce far different responses in different women.

That's why we can't chase symptoms alone. What is effective is to treat the underlying nature of menopause, which is hormonal imbalance instigated by declining estrogen levels. Estrogen apparently is the conductor of the orchestra and once estrogen departs the band starts playing different tunes.

Disruption in estrogen levels has been shown to cause everything from worry, anxiety, something they've been calling 'mental fog' and in some cases a sense of losing it mentally, of things slipping out of control to loss of sexual function. The spectrum of mental afflictions related to menopause ranges from non-existent to very worrisome and this mental-emotional aspect should be regarded as another of the individual aspects that makes every woman's experience of menopause unique. The possibility of sexual performance issues can't help but amplify the negative mental states that may already exist.

A common symptom that women tell me about is a sense of worry about their periods coming and going. They're worried about pregnancy and they're worried that the irregularity of skipped or changing periods may signal a deeper health crisis.

As the mind-body connection is so strong any change in the body results in a change in the mind. When a woman's mind is racing around with thoughts of undiagnosed illnesses lurking within, or unwanted pregnancy the mind can react in panic mode. As estrogen affects brain function any panic reaction that might once have been squashed by the power of a positive thought may now be magnified and elevated to large-scale importance. The mind, as we know has a tendency to repeat negative things over and over and when this tendency is paired with a brain that is experiencing unprecedented hormonal shifts the result is often an increase in anxiety and worry.

For some women this will be a difficult thing to deal with for others perhaps not so much. For a subset of menopausal women, the mental effects of this chemical imbalance will become a serious matter and require more serious treatments to rebalance the system.

The Doctor's Best Advice I can give to women, who are experiencing any level of mental affliction or sense of things coming unglued during the change of life, is to realize that this is almost surely due to hormonal imbalances. And hormonal imbalances can be corrected. The best way to keep the orchestra in tune and playing well together are a good Menopause Plan and a caring doctor.

BETH

When Beth first came to see me she was sixty-one. Her menopause started ten years earlier and she stayed in the care of her longtime internist who effectively treated her for high blood pressure, elevated cholesterol levels and occasional stomach problems for over twenty years.

When her internist retired she moved on to another doctor, then due to changes in medical insurance a third. It was this physician who referred her to me for a persistent problem that had troubled her on and off for a long time, bladder infections. Previous doctors had treated her with various antibiotics, yet the infections would always return.

After talking about her history and current medical issue I asked a series of questions to help diagnose her current state of health. "Since menopause, what treatments have you been using? Creams, herbals, lubrication, hormones, SSRI's?"

"I haven't been using anything." She replied.

"Are you sexually active?"

"Lord no," Beth said.

"Tell me about the bladder issues when did they start?"

"I'm thinking the first one was about age 55 and then maybe every year or so since then."

"When was the last time you had a visit with an ob-gyn?"

"When my last kid turned ten so I'd say twelve years, maybe more."

"Ok, why don't we do a physical exam and get a better picture of what's going on with your health?" I said.

Beth changed and was waiting for me on the exam table when I entered the room a few minutes later. I performed a routine examination and was able to gain insight to the underlying issues that Beth had presented. A short time later we were seated facing one another across my desk.

"Find anything interesting?" Beth asked as she shut off her phone and put it in her handbag.

"I found that you and I should talk a little bit about menopause, its effects on a woman's body and to formulate a Menopause Plan going forward."

"Menopause Plan? Really? I'm already through it. I'm finished with periods, hot flashes, emotional mood swings. It's over."

"I understand what you're saying as a personal experience, but menopause is a description of a process that starts with the first skipped period and continues for decades until the most senior of years. This is because menopause actually describes the time in a woman's life when her body is no longer producing the hormone estrogen. Estrogen is critical to good health. Without it a cascade of things happen to a woman's body. The first effects tend to be hot flashes, irritability and so on. Most of these symptoms diminish or disappear on their own given long enough. That's why many women consider menopause to be over, because the uncomfortable but transitory symptoms have abated."

Beth nodded her head in understanding, "Ok," she said.

"But estrogen's absence causes other problems as years go by. In your case the loss of estrogen had a common effect, the tissue that lines your vagina became thin or atrophic. As the older skin cells died fewer skin cells were taking their place. Layer by layer, year by year the skin was growing smoother, less elastic, less resilient. It went unnoticed perhaps because the change was so gradual that its effects became known only when the tissue became prone to infection. Gradually the pH balance shifts and the healthy bacteria that help to prevent infections diminish over time."

"Oh." Beth said.

"The reason you have been getting one infection after another, sometimes in the vagina, sometimes in the bladder is because the skin of your vagina is less healthy. We can treat the infections with antibiotics and they will go away for awhile, but each time we treat you in that manner we are still not getting at the root of the problem."

"Which is?"

"The effects of menopause," I said. "What I think we should do is to formulate a plan that will first treat your bladder infection, that's job one. Next, we should treat the genitourinary atrophy to reduce the chances of recurrence."

I wrote out a couple of prescriptions for Beth, one for a week-long course of antibiotics to treat the bladder issue. And a second prescription for a transdermal estrogen cream that she needed to apply daily for two weeks, then once a week. She made an appointment for six weeks later and I told her to contact me sooner if the bladder problem didn't clear up within five to seven days.

HANNAH

Hannah is a talented actor and has been working a "Survival job" as a waitress at an upscale seafood restaurant in Brooklyn for nearly fifteen years. Her day job affords her the chance to go out for auditions and roles her agent gets her without having the complications of a 9-5 job. In a way you've probably met Hannah before. That's because you've likely seen her as a character on Law and Order, sit-coms, Off-Broadway, Broadway and commercials like for Quaker Oats. She's a familiar face and a successful artist. She's also the mother of two grown kids (I delivered them both) and has been married to Stanley for twenty-seven years.

Our connection goes way back to when she was a new Mom seeking an obstetrician to help deliver her first child and I was a newly minted doctor eager to get my medical practice started. I asked about her first son as I opened Hannah's file, "Where's Kenny going?"

"Cornell, which he got a full scholarship to because of his baseball playing which I can only say thank God for because that place is break-the-bank expensive."

"What position does he play again?"

"First base. And Joey's going into the Marine Corps, he wants to go overseas," Hannah looked a little concerned as our eyes met.

"So, he's trying to kill Mama?" I said.

"Nothing new, he's the one with the motorcycle," She frowned.

"Oy!"

"Exactly. If that boy doesn't kill himself he'll kill me with a heart attack worrying about him," Hannah tugged at a kabala bracelet on her wrist.

"So they're out of the house?" I asked.

"Yup, I am officially an 'Empty Nester'."

"How's it going?"

"On what level?"

"Every level. How's Stanley?" I asked.

"Fine."

"How's your sex life?"

"Okay."

"That's what people say when their sex life is not so great," I said looking at her directly.

"I'm 53 years old, 'Sex life' is a description of history that's rolled on by."

"Lots of women still want to have sex at your age and much older," I said.

"Well you see that's the thing. I don't really want it anymore."

"Because of the dryness?"

"Possibly but lube seems to be working whenever I want to bother, it's not that. Let me put it this way. Take Brad Pitt as an example, ok?"

"Ok, Brad Pitt...? What?"

"You remember Thelma and Louise?"

"Yup," I said.

"Brad Pitt takes off his shirt. Great abs. Tight butt, cutest guy ever, right?"

"Right."

"It used to be all I had to do is look at his picture and I was ready, now I can watch the whole movie and it's a maybe."

"I get it. Are you and Stanley still good with each other?"

"Love him with all my heart."

"Ok, so let me ask a personal question," I began.

"Five minutes ago you had a speculum in my vagina, it doesn't get more personal than that, so go ahead, ask," Hannah said.

"When you were younger how was your sex life?"

"Before? It was good we enjoyed each other but you know with the kids and work and stuff, it got buried under a lot of other things. Lost its importance," Hannah said.

"Is Stanley still sexually interested?"

"Oh yeah, he's very annoying. Long story short, if I want to be nice we're talking oral, ok?" Hannah said.

"Alright so here's my thoughts, ready? It's time to rekindle the passion because my take is that sex has become about servicing Stanley more than about two people sharing an intimacy that has a deep bonding effect on a marriage. And I'm not hearing the word 'Orgasm' anywhere in this conversation, by the way. I'm not saying that you need to have sex with your husband on a regular basis, many women could let it go entirely but when something is lost like wanting to have the kind of sex that made you two really go for each other long ago, life gets less rich."

Hannah nodded in a sort of detached agreement.

"Here's what I think is going on. Once upon a time you couldn't wait to have sex with each other. You had a kid, then another. You both pursued careers. For years upon years life was about daycare, food on the table, stacks of bills, cleaning the house and dealing with piles of laundry. Bit by bit sex became a distant thing compared to the immediate things that needed attending to. There was no time, there was exhaustion when you finally hit the bed, there was a stress filled tomorrow waiting at the other end of the alarm clock. Kind of what happened?"

"Kinda."

"Your desire for sex died under the accumulated weight of living and the onset of menopause. I'm not saying you should return to sexual activity if you don't want to, but if you want to there's a way we can boost libido and sexual vibrancy. You can have great sex again after menopause, after kids and all that. Orgasms are good for you, your health your husband, your marriage, it's the hallmark of a strong vagina and a balanced life."

"I'm listening," Hannah said folding her hands in her lap.

And from there we launched a change to her Menopause Plan. It took two directions at the same time. One for the body and one for the mind. For the body we started with low dose hormone therapy that comes in a little soft plastic donut shape. Inserted into the vagina it releases estrogen in such tiny amounts it barely shows up in blood tests but works on the tissue that is its intended target.

The ring is an effective treatment for slowly rebuilding vaginal tissue. Soft, moist vaginal walls are important for enjoyable sex and are part of the solution for regaining sexual desire. As sex becomes more pleasurable and orgasms become easier to achieve and more frequent, desire inevitably arises. This is the mechanism we are trying to encourage from the body.

Caring for the mind is a separate issue. Sexual feelings and orgasms while certainly felt in the private parts actually occur only between the ears. When a pattern of routine sexual practices and routine sexual reactions, have been established over decades they can cause the mind to dull. Refreshing those pathways becomes key. "Yes," I told Hannah, "We're talking date night, sensual massage, Tantric practices, sex toys, lotions, candles, romance, erotica. Consider what works for you guys and do it, all the things younger couples might do and then some. Your vagina," I counseled her, "Can be made as vibrant as a thirty-year-old-woman's vagina. We can do that with medications and laser rejuvenation. But the real challenge is mental not medical. Let's fix the sexual issues that prevent libido from rising in you and you work on the things that make libido rise."

"Masturbation?" She asked.

"Absolutely," I replied. And there we left it. A program had been formed and I knew that the next time we got together Hannah and I would be having an interesting conversation about what was working and what could still use a little work. I didn't let Hannah know, because we'd covered enough ground in one visit, but I had a few tricks up my sleeve in case we needed a boost later on.

Physician Heal Thyself

My own experience with menopause started in my fifty-fifth year when I was struck by an illness that hit me so powerfully and swiftly that before I knew it I was lying on the bathroom floor trying to stay conscious enough to call for help. Somehow I did and the next memory that I have of that day is coming to in my beloved Lenox Hill Hospital. All around me were familiar faces. I'd known the Emergency Room Physician for ten years. The Head Nurse was my patient. I knew the Registered Nurses, orderlies and housekeepers by name. I knew many of these people's families and had helped some of them with medical issues over the years. No one was used to seeing me lying on a gurney in need of a doctor's care, especially me.

The pain was so powerful that the Emergency Room doctor gave me a shot of morphine just so that I could communicate enough to help them diagnose me. The questions came fast.

"Do you have a heart condition?"

"No."

"History of stroke?"

"No."

"High blood pressure?"

"No."

"Are you on any drugs or alcohol?"

"No."

"When was your last period and are you taking estrogen?"

"Over five years ago and no I'm not taking estrogen"

And at that moment I became aware of the presence of my best friend and fellow obstetrician-gynecologist Janet, who I completed my residency with and have known for over twenty years. Janet was making hospital rounds when she heard I was in the ER and came running.

She leaned in close, her face a mask of worry and concern and she said in a voice filled with incredulity, "What do you mean you're not taking estrogen!?!" Which made me laugh because that definitely was not what was wrong with me. Women don't fall down unconscious and go into shock because their estrogen levels are too low, the ER Doc was asking because of the remote possibility of a complication of pregnancy.

The Emergency Room doctor was a former colonel in the U.S. Army and he shot Janet a look that could've frozen water. As their eyes met he said to her, "Please leave now." And she did, slinking off just far enough to stay out of the Big Doc's way but close enough to keep an eye on me.

My fifty-fifth year had barely started and no one knew if I was dying. My husband was out of town and rushing back to be by my side. Friends and colleagues in the hospital where I'd spent over twenty years of my life surrounded me. As the full dose of painkillers hit me, I drifted off to an odd dream state where Janet was chasing me with a speculum and a small donut made of plastic.

CHAPTER 2

THE FIRST GOLDEN AGE FOR OLDER WOMEN

THERE HAS NEVER been a better time to be an older woman than the age we now live in. Women these days had the advantages of good health care when they were younger, birth control when they were in their reproductive years and sound medical treatment, as they got older. It wasn't always this way.

The History of Menopause deserves only a few words. There was the Age of Early Death (Self-explanatory), the Age of Only Herbals (10,000 B.C. to 1947), the Age of Massive Overtreatment (1960's-2002) and the Golden Age of Menopause (2015-present).

Women's health through the ages was always fragile due to multiple pregnancies and reproductive complications. Any infection could be a death sentence or a lifetime of pain. Many deliveries could easily result in death for the mother, baby or both. Add in the problems of war, food insecurity, bad water, cholera epidemics, plagues, flu, untreated medical conditions and the end result was unavoidable. Women died young. Menopause therefore wasn't widely experienced and treatments for it remained unchanged for thousands of years.

The best of times for older women began when low dose, targeted Hormone Replacement Therapy (HRT) became available. This was a groundbreaking development because the previous generation of almost exclusively male doctors had been treating menopause simplistically. Instead of precise targeting of medications they carpet-bombed women's bloodstreams with systemic hormone replacements.

Their reasoning went like this; women experience menopause due to low estrogen therefore if you flood their bodies with estrogen menopause is cured. The results were catastrophic for the health of some women and that is why Hormone Replacement Therapy fell into disfavor. The carpet- bombing approach to menopause yielded death and disease for some women and the media in turn carpet-bombed the idea of Hormone Replacement Therapy until the entire concept was burnt to a cinder.

Destroying Hormone Replacement Therapy as a viable treatment for menopause created an entirely new set of issues. Large numbers of women born in the Baby Boom generation were entering menopause. For the first time in history women were independent, educated, sexually free, with careers and choices about family planning, marriage and divorce.

As millions of women approached their fifties all at the same time they discovered that there were no effective treatments for most menopausal symptoms, especially the most severe ones. Neither doctors nor patients wanted anything to do with hormone replacements and that left only herbals, lubricants and medications for sleeplessness as remedies.

At this same moment in time, and due to the same large historical forces that gave us the Baby Boomers, a large number of women obstetrician-gynecologists were earning their degrees and beginning medical practice. The previous generation of ob-gyn's were nearly all men and their ways and manners did not reflect the sweeping changes in both attitude and behavior of the new age. The swagger of the John Wayne World War II era male doctors at the end of their careers did not mesh well with the Woodstock era women doctors beginning their careers. Menopause was only one of the grounds for disagreement.

Out of this cauldron of change, both pharmaceutical and generational, came an amazing new array of medications and treatments. Which from a historical perspective, arose at just the right time. The Baby Boomers were now almost all passing fifty, many were knocking on the door of sixty and few of them had been given estrogen replacement.

The result was catastrophe. Vaginal atrophy that had been greatly reduced in their mother's generation (With many bad side effects) by the bombardment method was now back again. Most women were now suffering from the same type of menopause their grandmothers had lived through.

The difference between them and their grandmothers was that many had a sex-positive attitude toward life and they wanted sex to continue. They'd been encouraged from a young age to think of themselves as sexual people. To have fun, experiment, have orgasms, establish relationships. The culture of eternal youth that America embraces also embraces a notion that sex and interested partners will always be a part of a natural life.

And that was the catastrophe that began to ripple through many women's lives. For them sex was a memory. The need for it faded over the years and in a subtle, gradual way that went unnoticed, they stopped being sexual women. The fact that it was caused by estrogen depletion was either unknown or ignored. The gradual and subtle nature of its progression made its advance practically unnoticeable and bit by bit sexual energy faded for many women until sexual activity itself became a bit of history.

The fading of sex into the sands of time might still be the main experience of women as they enter menopause except for two unprecedented changes in the world of menopause treatments. One of these groundbreakers comes from Big Pharma and the other from advances in high technology. The pharmaceutical breakthrough came in the late nineties when low dose estrogen therapy became available in a wide range of product types. Some were creams, others were patches and still others came as insert-able devices. The combination of different types and doses of medications allowed physicians to individualize the treatment for each woman.

Now menopause treatments did not have to be one size fits all. Localized or topical therapies could safely direct the treatment to the effected areas of the vagina. The skin cells that needed estrogen could be supplied with estrogen by direct contact, not from absorption through the systemic blood supply.

This is hugely significant because the previous forms of Hormone Replacement Therapy were a total body experience when only a pin-prick was needed. As a result, the dosages needed to treat damaged tissues were miniscule compared to the previous generation of estrogen medications. Bad health outcomes dropped dramatically until they became statistically insignificant.

The new methods of treating menopause had been determined and finally doctors could offer significant help as women began to experience symptoms including painful sex and vaginal atrophy.

Or so we would like to think. In reality what happened was that both physicians and patients largely ignored the scientific results. Hormone Replacement Therapy of either high or low dose had been taken out of the playbook due to the earlier illnesses and the crushing media onslaught of a decade earlier. Even though times had changed and medical treatment had advanced, the practice of menopause medicine was right where it had been in Grandma's time. Physicians preferred not to use it out of fear of causing harm and patients avoided it out of fear of being harmed.

In the past few years, doctors began to make women's sexual health from young adulthood to menopause a subspecialty within obstetrics-gynecology. Women doctors who had been in the first wave of medical students and residencies were now becoming senior doctors and also senior women. The new generation of women doctors started to enter menopause themselves and somewhere in this stew of feminist advancement, pharmaceutical inventions and the emergence of practical treatments, menopause began to be something that could be effectively treated.

It is probably not a coincidence that this advanced focus on treating menopause arose when women physicians were facing the change of life themselves. Men had always run the show regarding women's health and now women had a seat at the table for the first time in history and they needed ways to treat their own menopause.

KATHERINE

Katherine came back a month later as we had planned to talk about how her treatment with the low dose estrogen cream was going. After we said our hellos and spent a few moments in small talk Katherine said, "He didn't leave."

"Who didn't leave?" I asked.

"Timmy, the guy I tried to have sex with. I figured after that night we were finished."

"But?"

"But he stuck around. I told him what was going on and told him it wasn't him, it wasn't a technique thing and no, he wasn't too big for me. It was a minor medical thing, it wasn't an STD and I promised him that I'd be good to go pretty soon."

"Alright great, so how are you feeling?" I asked.

"Better. Not a whole lot but with lube I think it'll be ok. It's kind of hard for me to know so before I let Timmy go all the way again I was thinking you should take a look under the hood."

"My thought exactly," I said and we headed to the exam room. What I saw was good. The vaginal atrophy had abated, the skin had indeed improved and the treatment had thus far been successful. For now, in the narrow timeframe of thirty days we really couldn't have hoped for a better outcome.

Menopause treatment I reminded Katherine lasts as long as menopause itself. As time passes the effects of menopause will change and the treatments required to maintain a state of vaginal health will also change as a result. Treating menopause means adjusting treatments as menopause itself changes over time. But for now, we were hitting all the right notes.

"Alright Doc," She said as I completed my exam, "The suspense is killing me. Am I good to go?"

"Yes. I'm happy to report you have much better tissue growth and unless he's truly 'Too big'…?"

Katherine smiled and shook her head no.

"I think you should be able to have vaginal intercourse without pain or discomfort."

"Thank you Dr. Fein, I'll let you know how it works out."

I was hoping that in another month when she returned for a follow-up I would hear about the next installment of the Katherine and Timmy story but only two days later she sent me a selfie of herself with a big smile and a thumbs up gesture. I couldn't help but notice that her hair was tousled and her pajama top was inside out.

DYNAMIC & UNIQUE

Men are more steady-state creatures than women are. Their hormone levels tend to be more stable. If we were to plot a graph of the levels in their bloodstream through the day or even over years, it would remain kind of flat. We would not see the continual fluctuations that are typical and normal for women.

Women are dynamic creatures by the very design of their bodies and exist in an ever-changing pattern of flux. This pattern of hormonal expression is unique to each woman and the regularity of its fluctuations becomes normal for that woman. It's as if a baseline of cyclic changes is established and is maintained specific to the individual. The body and mind working together appear to form internal strategies to cope with this life-long pattern, in effect making it a normal operating condition.

Until menopause. Then everything goes out of kilter because the body is no longer making certain hormones. We know that estrogen is not the only factor in what we call "Menopause." There are at least eight other hormones that effect each other and then are effected themselves by the interaction. The dynamism of menopause has its genesis in the dynamism of hormonal interactions, the complexities of which are ever changing. When they are in balance, like in reproductive age women, the complex interactions are the foundation for both menstrual cycle regulation and even the basis for fertility. As the hormonal levels reconfigure themselves in menopause, the mechanism that once established stability from a chaotic process can be overwhelmed.

During menopause both the actual and relative levels of hormones fluctuate in an unprecedented fashion. The timing and sequence of changes appears to be unique to the individual and somewhat unpredictable. The body that once knew how to create stability from volatility may not know how to accomplish that task any longer. Therefore, treating menopause includes adjusting hormonal balances. Smoothing out the spikes and troughs makes for a smoother ride over the bumps and furrows of menopause. This process is called "Ramping" and is used to prevent the worst effects of menopause from asserting themselves.

Ramping should begin as soon as a woman begins to have symptoms that cause distress and may continue throughout her menopause. Beginning treatment early allows for precise dosages of medications to be applied when they will be most effective. This gives the best results and generates the longest lasting positive effects.

Many women seek treatment only when symptoms like sexual issues become a real problem and that indicates they waited too long to begin their Menopause Plan. Ideally the plan a woman should be following begins as the first hormonal shifts begin. This is the point at which the standard volatility a woman experienced from post-puberty through her reproductive years has now ended.

At this point if left untreated, hormones may now begin to rage out of control. By addressing the effects of menopause at fifty or sixty years old instead of earlier, women may lose the opportunity for the best possible outcome while they experience the symptoms caused by the extremes of hormonal shifts. Regulating hormonal extremes offers women a way to establish a new normal as things gradually regain a new balance.

Menopause no longer means that sexual vibrancy inevitably diminishes. With proper planning and health care sexuality can continue in an unbroken chain from young adulthood to the most senior of years. A woman with a good plan for her menopause armed with a good doctor for a coach should experience menopause as a gentle turning of the wheel instead of the beginning of the end for her sexuality.

SOFIA

Sofia returned for an office visit six months after our last conversation for a matter unrelated to pre-menopause. Her Pap smear results were slightly abnormal and the correct protocol for her was to repeat the test in six months. An abnormal Pap usually does not mean that a patient has cancer but does have an increased risk so the situation should be monitored closely and at regular intervals.

"Hello Sofia, how are you? Are you well?" I asked as I shook her hand hello.

"Hello Dr. Fein. I feel good."

"Still running?" I asked.

"Oh yeah, I did the Run For the Cure 10k in Central Park last week."

"Me too. I think I finished last, what was your time?"

"Thirty one minutes, thirty seconds." Sofia said.

"You're fast, I did it in a little under an hour."

"That's pretty good, how often do you run?"

"Couple of times a week schedule allowing," I said as she sat on the exam table.

"So I have a question about diabetes."

"Yes?" I said as I put on my gloves and sat down to do her exam.

"How often should I get that checked?"

"The A1C test results were normal. There's only a very small chance you'll ever develop diabetes, so I'd put that worry mostly out of your mind. As a precautionary thing we should check again in a year or two but we need to watch the Paps every six months depending on what this next report shows. Anything else going on? Itching? Burning? Odor? Stress overload? Any stomachaches? Are you pooping every day?"

"No problems. Stress comes and goes, I deal. My stomach's fine and I poop twice a day usually."

"Excellent. Any burning when you urinate?"

"Nope."

"Are you sexually active? Are you in a relationship? Any worries about STD's?"

"No. No. No."

"Okay just try to relax for a minute," I said as I placed the speculum as gently as I could to get the sample to send to the lab for her Pap test.

"So, last time we spoke you had irregular periods. How's that going anything you'd like to discuss?"

"Same as last time. No real changes I can see." Sofia said.

"Great. What about the hot flashes?"

"They suck and are getting a little worse but I've been using black cohosh."

"How's it working?"

"Okay," Sofia said, "How do I look inside?" She asked as I completed my exam and signaled she should sit up.

"Your cervix looks fine I'm not worried and we'll have the Pap result in a week or two. But I'm starting to see some signs of vaginal atrophy, which as we spoke about will slowly get worse each year. Remember we spoke about estrogen replacement?"

"Yes very well, I'm still opposed."

"Totally ok with me," I said, "I just want to keep you informed of what's going on down there."

"Are there any new herbal treatments for the atrophy?"

"I wish there were. Herbal remedies work better for hot flashes and mood swings than to treat the vaginal dryness. At the moment the best treatment we have is low dose Hormone Replacement Therapy for the stage of menopause you are currently in. In the future you might want to consider vaginal laser rejuvenation treatment if you develop more severe symptoms. The laser thing is done without any hormones just laser light. For the time being let's try a non-hormonal moisturizer that comes as a vaginal suppository, you use it once or twice a week and it will help slow down the changes from the lower estrogen levels you're experiencing." I rummaged through a cabinet and handed Sofia a sample tube.

She looked it over, read the label and handed it back to me, Sofia crossed her arms over her chest, "Too Big Pharma for me to be comfortable with it, is it ok if I don't?"

"Absolutely. If you're fine with that, I'm fine with that," I said, "Unfortunately we don't have an organic natural substance or cream yet that works or I would've suggested it. If as time goes by, you develop symptoms that make you uncomfortable remember the door is always open. Just come in and we'll figure out the best way to tweak your Menopause Plan. For now, I'm confident you have the plan that's best for you and like we've talked about, as your menopause changes, we can change the plan as well."

Sofia and I spoke about other things for a couple of minutes, we're both Mets fans and they had just won a 10 inning game the night before. We said goodbye until we'd meet again in about six months. Her most recent Pap came back about a week later and Sofia was doing fine the results were stable.

MADELINE

It was one of those weird things that happen sometimes and you can't really explain it, so you just let it go. I read a story in Art News about Madeline's husband Murray donating some paintings to the Metropolitan Museum and I was like, that's nice. Then when I got to the office I saw that Madeline was first on the schedule for that day. Weird.

"Oh no I was mad as hell!" She said when I told her I'd seen the article. "The Chagall was mine, I was very emphatic that I wanted it to stay right where it was. After we're gone I could care less, but until that day arrives, the Chagall was supposed to stay on the wall in Amagansett and that was that!"

"So, what happened?" I asked.

"Some slick girl curator from the Met charmed him and he fell for it. How can such a brilliant man be such a colossal oaf?"

"Wow. I remember the Chagall."

"Oaf!"

We both looked at one another for a long moment, "I'm assuming this did nothing good for the emotional surges?" I asked.

"Is it that obvious?" She said with a wry smile, "I thought I was hiding it well." We both laughed.

"How did the herbal supplement work?"

"On a scale of one to ten?" She asked, "A two."

"Mindfulness Based Stress Reduction?"

"Actually I like the guy you recommended and I'm sticking with that. It helps but I'd put it as a six out of ten. On a good day."

"How about Yoga, a daily fitness routine? Were you able to go with that?" I asked.

"Oh yes. I joined a gym, I found a Yoga guru and I learned two things. I hate the gym. I hate the Yoga studio. Just the smell of those places makes me want to gag."

"Alright I hear you. I still want to urge you to find something, anything that gets you up doing some kind of exercise everyday, walking vigorously, swimming…? Madeline shook her head no.

"Biking?" She shot me an 'Are you kidding?' look.

"Pole dancing?" I offered.

"I appreciate the attempt at humor but the fact is it's not me. I'm built for heels and lunch at the Carlyle. If they invent a sport that combines those two, I'm in."

"Ok, then let's try something that works but is less organic than the other stuff. It's a medication."

"A pill? Hurray! Hip, hip hurray!"

"You seem receptive."

"I've always liked a good pill."

"I'm going to leave that one alone for the time being. Let's talk about the kind that don't get you high."

"Oh alright," Madeline said feigning disappointment.

"I think the pill that will work best for you, is what's called an SSRI or selective serotonin reuptake inhibitor. For menopause treatment it comes in very low dosages and has two benefits for your condition. The first is that it will reduce hot flashes and mood swings without any hormones that could aggravate your fibroid problem. Second a common minor side effect is it may make you a little drowsy so if you take it before bed it should help you sleep. When it works well, which it usually does, women tell me 'I just feel like myself again' just be patient, give it a few weeks to work."

"Valium is very good for mood swings," Madeline offered, "I read it on the internet which is the most unimpeachable of sources."

"Nice try. Here's a prescription for the SSRI, call me if have any questions and let's get together again in a month. Stay with the MBSR. How's your alcohol use by the way?"

"Never touch the stuff."

"No, really."

"Fine, I'll cut back." Madeline put on her tailored overcoat and walked down the hallway to the exit.

I called out, "Try and forgive Murray!" She balled up her fists at the mention of her husband's name. "He gave away the Chagall!" She yelled before stomping off. A moment later I heard a very small, muffled voice coming through the walls, "Oaf!!" and then the sound of a door slamming.

LAURA AND PATTY

Laura and Patty are a same sex couple I've been seeing for over ten years. They first met as college roommates and at some point between their freshman and sophomore years they stopped dating boys and starting dating each other. After years of living together they tied the knot as soon as gay marriage became legal and have been happily married ever since. They preferred to come together for their appointments and it was always nice to see them again.

"Doc!" They both said at the same time and gave me a hug hello.

"Hey Ladies!"

"So, let's start with you Patty. What's new? How are you feeling? Are you in good health?"

"Ah no," She said.

"Bleeding issues," Laura said.

"For you or Patty?" I asked.

"Me," Patty said.

"Ok, can you describe the bleeding for me?" I asked.

"It started near Thanksgiving and you know we're both forty five years old now so I figure irregular bleeding, menopause. You know no big deal. Like I heard this happens and now, so here it is. Kind of on schedule." Patty said.

"But it didn't stop," Laura continued, "The bleeding was heavier than Patty normally gets in a period. Then it stopped and started. And that's when I started to get a little scared."

"So we came in," Patty said.

"Ok, I got the picture. Patty do you have any other symptoms of menopause?"

"Irregular bleeding is about it."

"Laura, how about you?"

"Oh me? Well, I got the whole pantheon of woman troubles, from night sweats to hot flashes. No excessive bleeding though."

"How would you describe your periods?"

"Lighter than before."

"Alrighty then, let's take a look. Who wants to hop up first?" I asked. They exchanged a quick glance with one another and then Patty took the first turn while Laura held her hand. Then they reversed positions and within a few minutes I knew everything that a physical exam could reveal in this single visit. Treatment would require a diagnostic test and a return appointment because we needed more information to work with before we could make a plan.

Laura and Patty came back about two weeks later when the blood tests were in and the results of a sonogram had been evaluated. We settled around my desk in the too cramped office, piled with papers and memos.

"So?" Patty asked.

I took the sonogram out of a folder and used a pencil as a pointer to show what I was explaining to Patty, Laura leaned in close to get a better view, "It looks like you have an endometrial polyp that is a growth that attaches to the uterine lining. Most people have heard of polyps as in polyps in your colon which can be cancer or precancerous but uterine polyps are almost always benign. We could just take a biopsy in the office to confirm. But in your case it should come out because it's causing you to bleed and it's serious enough that we should schedule a procedure to remove it."

"Are you talking about surgery?" Laura asked in alarm, which made Patty sit up in alarm.

"Yes we need to do it in an operating room under general anesthesia at the hospital. The procedure itself will take about thirty minutes. You'll need a few hours recuperation and then you can go home. That day you may feel a little dizzy or nauseous and some cramping and bleeding is expected for a week or two. Take it easy, come in for a checkup in about two weeks, then you can go back to all activities." I said scribbling notes in Patty's chart. "Polyps can grow back so we'll have to keep watch but you shouldn't continue to have excessive bleeding."

Laura looked at Patty in deep concern and then turned toward me, "Is this what you call Dilation and Curettage?"

"Yes, that would be the technical term for doing the various things needed to remove the growth. Usually I use a little camera to look around first and we call that a Hysteroscopy."

"Is there any alternative to surgery? Nutritional changes, anything?" Patty asked.

"I wish there were. Unfortunately the only way to stop the bleeding is to remove the growth. It can't get better on its own, only worse. It's a real health concern if it's not addressed and my advice is to get it seen to as soon as you can."

"Ohmigod," Laura said softly to herself.

"It'll be ok," Patty said.

"Yes, it will definitely be ok. It's a common problem and a routine procedure. You'll get back to normal activities quickly. I'll give you some information so you'll know more about what's coming up then call the office and we'll get you scheduled? Ok?"

They looked at one another and nodded yes in unison.

"And now let's talk about Laura," I said.

"You're scaring me."

"Please relax and unclench. Patty will be fine. And there's nothing much the matter with you we can't treat easily. So here's the findings. You have begun pre-menopause."

"Ah, I thought so," Laura said looking down. They both became quiet for a moment.

"Can I ask a question?" Patty said.

"Of course, anything," I replied.

"Before the bleeding started when things were still pretty normal, I noticed a change in Laura that I wanted to ask you about," Patty said. "I don't know how to put this because its kind of embarrassing and Laura's not going to like I brought this up here." She paused and took a breath, "But our sex life is going downhill fast."

"Really?" Laura said turning toward Patty.

"We used to have sex a few times a week, then once a week, then a couple times a month. I'm like into it, ready to get something started and Laura just doesn't turn on."

"Really? Again, really?" Laura said again, folding her arms across her chest.

I decided to jump in, "Alright, I actually have something to offer here and Laura I know this is a difficult place and everything to be going into this, but it's also a really good place in some ways. So here's the news, everything you're experiencing is consistent with menopause. Your hormones are going crazy and what do hormones control?"

"Sex stuff," Laura replied.

"Yes and so, the hot flashes and the low libido, the sleeplessness and sweats are because of low estrogen. Patty is observing the side effects of menopauses worst and longest lasting effect, vaginal atrophy. That I hasten to add is highly treatable. But because of it sex drive suffers."

"Vaginal atrophy," She said to herself softly as if in disbelief.

"A harsh word or phrase, I know," I said. "But what is, is what is. Menopause is the source of your problems. And modern medicine has a solution. At forty-five years old you're young enough that Hormone Replacement Therapy, the kind that is safe, the same kind that women doctors use on themselves, will help enormously. That's for the hot flashes and so on. For the vaginal atrophy here's another strategy that we can add. It's the vaginal ring and or estrogen cream. The ring is like a small, soft donut impregnated with low dose estrogen that stays in the vagina. This slowly releases tiny amounts of hormones exactly where they are needed and works directly to improve the dry skin allowing for the regrowth of healthy tissue. Together with a topical cream you can apply if you want or need to, things will start to feel better in no time. Here's the best part, by starting now you'll have an easier time going through menopause and a healthier vagina for the rest of your life. Better sex too."

Laura and Patty both followed Doctor's Best Advice and we removed Patty's polyp about two weeks later. She recovered quickly and the bleeding improved. Laura's Menopause Plan was very effective. The hot flashes, sleeplessness etc. diminished greatly. A subsequent checkup after the medications had been used for a month revealed that things were going very well. Her vaginal skin had become softer and moister. There was abundant new tissue growth signaling that soon her sex drive should start rebounding.

Both Patty and Laura saw changes in their bodies as a result of aging and for each of them it was a different experience. Patty first thought that her menopause was asserting itself as irregular bleeding, when in fact the bleeding was caused by a medical issue, requiring a surgical solution. Luckily they didn't wait any longer and didn't make a common mistake many women make that is to assume that all changes in bleeding are attributable to menopause. They frequently are but sometimes they are not and only a doctor can tell the difference.

Laura was equally as lucky as Patty in seeking timely doctor's advice. By coming up with a Menopause Plan while she was still in the earliest stages, effective treatments will yield both a positive impact early with lower doses and longer lasting beneficial effects later. It is better whenever possible to treat menopause early rather than wait for symptoms to make life miserable let alone suffer the loss of sexual vibrancy.

JULIE

Julie is forty-one years old and the married mother of three small children ranging in ages from three to twelve. She's a stay-at-home Mom dedicating herself to the kids and her husband Jay who she met about fifteen years ago. Jay's an architect who works on big projects like skyscrapers and stadiums. Which was how he met Julie. She was working as a junior architect at a company that handles the steelwork for massive projects and they started interacting professionally, hit it off personally and eventually got hitched. I became their obstetrician and delivered all three of the kids, so Julie and I had a long history together.

Jay worked with big name architects usually referred to as "Starchitects" as their right hand man. The Starchitect would draw the building, its designs and features and Jay would fill in the blanks and interact with the construction companies who actually built the thing. Julie would sometimes invite me along for a tour of the unfinished building and we'd put on hard hats and follow Jay around as he pointed out what would be built in the near future. It was thrilling to see the skeleton frame of a skyscraper turn into a finished building and then about a year later be filled with life and activity, restaurants serving people and office workers rushing around. My favorite was the Hearst Tower on 57th Street that rose from the center of a 1930's low rise building into the sky.

"Tracey!"

"Julie!" We hugged for a quick second and I gave her a good looking over. "You look tired," I said.

"That's what people tell you when they mean to say 'You look old'."

"No, I meant to say you look tired. Are you sleeping well?"

Julie sighed and sat down heavily, "I'll sleep when I'm dead."

"Which will come sooner if you're not sleeping well. Sleeping is really important for good health. What is it the kids?" She shook her head and clammed up. I figured that maybe something would come out of the exam so I talked to her about an architecture and art exhibit that was going on at Cooper Union and after awhile, we shifted to medical things.

"I think I'm going through menopause," She said at last.

"No you're not. Why would you think that?" I said. She was a perfectly healthy forty-one year old woman. Julie was still getting her periods with regularity so there was only slight if any diminishment of estrogen in her body. She was not in menopause.

"It's the symptoms. I'm irritable. I can't sleep. And if Jay even thinks of having sex with me I pretend I'm an iceberg until he leaves me alone. Menopause." Julie said making a palms-up gesture.

"No, not menopause," I repeated, "There's lots of reasons for all three of those symptoms you told me about; loss of interest in sex, irritability, sleeplessness. And we can offer treatments for all three but the reason you have these symptoms is still a little mysterious to me. Do you mind if I play Sherlock Holmes here for a minute?" She nodded yes and so I continued onward, "How are things between you and Jay?"

"We get along. I love him. We're good together with the kids."

"Is there anything about him sexually that is turning you off?"

She nodded no with a shoulder shrug attached, "It's me, he's perfectly attractive. I'm sure if he did Tinder someone would do him."

"Ok, are the kids too much? Stress overload?"

"I'm good with the Mommy thing, they're fun. They make me smile everyday and the three year old makes me laugh just to look at her."

"Ok, good. You can't sleep. You're irritable but it's not the kids. And the perfect husband is still committed and home but you're not into him," I said.

"What's your diagnosis?"

"Actually I'm still probing you for clues. When did you first notice the loss of sex drive, irritability and so on. Did they all come together? Can you peg it with a date?

Julie frowned and sighed deeply, "August 1ˢᵗ this year."

"Wow I was thinking you'd say late winter, or something more general. What happened August 1ˢᵗ?" I asked.

"Joshua and Marley moved in and on that day the beginning of the end started for me."

"Ah, go on," I said resting my chin on my hand, "Who are they?"

"Joshua is Jay's father, my father-in-law and Marley is his third wife fifty seven years old. And they're living in the bedroom down the hall from the master with Debbie and her sister relocated to what was once

47

the study. Long story short, Joshua got fired in the Big Crunch when he was almost sixty no one would give him a job, he burned through savings, the IRA, sold the house. Complete shipwreck and they washed ashore in my living room."

"And how are you getting along?"

"Joshua is a sweetie, I can see why Jay came out so good. But Marley is how should I put this? A parasite and a bitch? Yeah that's it. I mean she moves in and on top of Jay and three kids I'm now her maid? I mean I clean her bathroom for God's sake! And what do I get from it? An angry, unhinged woman who bitches constantly and tells me why I'm stupid twenty times a day." Julie stopped talking and her face was now drawn with anger, every muscle in her body seemed to have tightened up at the same moment.

"I think I have a diagnosis," I said. "First, you and Jay need to dump the kids for a three-day weekend and go someplace alone. If you're not having sexual relations with passion after three days with a guy hot enough to score on Tinder, we'll talk again. Next, you yourself are perfectly healthy. Lastly, I do believe on further analysis that menopause is in fact the heart of what is going on here. But it's not your menopause, its Marley's. She's driving you crazy from stress because her hormones are driving her crazy. Is she seeing someone to treat her menopause?"

"She doesn't have health care. She's too young for Medicare and can't afford the deductibles on Obamacare."

"Send her to me and then we'll get you healed up. One condition though, you and Jay go on a second honeymoon and let Joshua and Marley babysit. If things don't improve you come back no later than a month from now and we work harder to get you back to a happy Julie. Promise?" I said holding out my pinkie. Julie took her pinkie and hooked it around mine and we shook.

"Promise," She said.

I talked to her about exercise; Yoga and MBSR because these things will help balance her mind and her body and help reduce Marley's toxic effects upon her. As her mind and body strengthen up, her coping mechanisms will also become stronger and more resilient, these are often just as effective as medications, which if at all possible should be avoided. The fewer medications one takes, the better.

Marley came in for treatment a week later and I helped her formulate a Menopause Plan that would help her feel better. Hopefully, I reasoned, as her symptoms improved so would Julie's and the difficulties that menopause was presenting in her household would soon melt away. Or become tolerable. I'm not a miracle worker.

TRACEY

The funny thing about a sudden crushing illness that makes you unconsciousness and sends you into shock is that you're in denial that it's happening until you're laid out on the floor unable to move. Then it starts to sink in. Like a swimmer underwater your consciousness bubbles to the surface, looks around and then submerges again into unconsciousness.

When I made it to the Emergency Room all I knew was that I was extremely ill and at first I wasn't the only one who thought it was a heart attack. In quick order they hooked me up to an EKG machine and took a look at the printout. Steady. No arrhythmia. Nothing that indicated heart trouble. My husband arrived and held my hand and did as much as he could to comfort me as various techs and doctors shot something into me or took blood out of me. Before I knew it, in a hazy blur of details I was being transported through the hospital hallways I'd walked ten thousand times before. But now all I saw were banks of overhead fluorescent lights as they wheeled me toward Radiology.

The CAT machine or CAT scan is a common sight to doctors, we've all ordered these tests thousands of times. So when I lifted my head to see where I was, it was someplace real familiar. But the experience became very fresh when they handed me a glass full of some vile radio-active dye laced drink and said, "Drink it all down."

I took a sip and retched. "Mint," I thought, "I hate mint." I couldn't even handle a glass of water and the next fifteen minutes were a battle zone between what I needed to do and what my body would allow me to tolerate. Eventually the witches brew made its way into my system and they wheeled me into the room with the machine that would scan my insides to detect what was wrong.

Somewhere within the thousands of images this amazing machine would produce, I hoped someone would find something they could diagnose and treat. As the CAT machine's flatbed moved me forward millimeter-by-millimeter to do its scan, I silently prayed this was just going to be a bad day and not a bad year. Or worse.

Sex and the Brain

Sexual vibrancy is something that most women wish to maintain all their lives. It is frequently a regular activity and source of pleasure but it also helps bond two people together in a loving relationship. Its absence in a person's life can be difficult to adjust to.

As we've seen, The Menopause Plan addresses the changes over long periods of time that leads to the inevitable deterioration of women's sexual functioning. The Plan itself is a guide for preventing problems from arising and for treating problems as they develop. The end goal is an uninterrupted life of joyful sexuality and good overall health. Menopause is no longer the beginning of the end of being a sexual woman, with proper treatment, sexual activity no longer has an end date. For women who are not sexually active, maintaining vaginal health remains an important part of maintaining overall health.

The complexities of women's sexuality are not limited to hormonal balances alone. Sex is also tied to brain functions. Neuroscientists have been mapping human brain activity with imaging machines for over a decade now and their findings are highly informative.

The first fun fact to emerge from the labs of the neuroscientists is that they were able to recruit nine women who agreed to stimulate themselves to orgasm while undergoing an MRI scan. The concept was to map a woman's brain during orgasm to see what regions lit up and what went dark. They flip booked the images into a movie and it gives a 3-D representation of a woman during orgasm. You can watch it if you want on YouTube.

Orgasms, it has often been noted happen primarily in a person's head despite all appearances to the contrary. The surge of pleasurable chemicals and powerful rushes of happy warm feelings are the result of various chemicals being released that cause different brain areas to be stimulated. Some of the areas like those that make us aware of our surroundings are temporarily shut down and others are made highly energetic making us aware of deep pleasure. In a way it is a consciousness changing experience that lifts the brain from one state of cognition to a very different one.

For orgasms in women to occur there must be correct stimulation of both the body and the mind. There is a deep connection between the two and any interruption in the chemical signaling between them results in a change of neurotransmitter responses in the brain. The chemical responses arise from the physical stimulation of nerve cells controlling sexual feelings and eventual orgasm. Any health issue that prevents stimulation of nerve endings in the sexual regions prevents the brain signals from being initiated.

That is what occurs with vaginal atrophy. The cells are damaged and cannot convey the signals to the brain that are needed to create feelings of sexual attraction, stimulation and orgasm. The brain-body connection is absolute. Any interruption in the nerve endings of the body that causes a reduced production of sex chemicals in the brain results in an interruption of the sexual response.

The second interesting fact to arise from the mapping of the brain's sexual response is in regards to the two pathways to orgasm, vaginal and clitoral. It's been known for a long time that women are more likely to reach climax as a result of multiple areas being stimulated at the same time. Some women can have an orgasm from a single point of stimulation while for others this is difficult to achieve.

Neuroscience has contributed some clarity to this issue. It seems to be a question of wiring. Nerve endings fan out within the skin to create a web of sensors that pick up various stimulations and convey them back to the brain. Some of these networks of nerves are more tightly packed and more numerous in number in some areas than in others and they are also specific to what type of information they convey.

Nerve cells in the clitoris and walls of the vagina relay sexual information to the brain but they may not be wired in identical patterns either in relation to one another or from woman to woman. Some women on an anatomical level may have more nerve endings in their clitoris than other women. Some may have fewer. The most common route to orgasm is through multiple stimulation of both the clitoris and vagina. However, if a woman has the correct configuration, single region stimulation alone may be sufficient, it's all about the wiring that connects the body to the brain.

The MRI scans of women having orgasms showed that at least eighty different regions of the brain become activated through the sequence of arousal, stimulation, climax and afterglow. Additional regions such as the prefrontal cortex may show different types of responses depending if the woman is controlling her own orgasm or if there is a partner involved.

As stimulation begins to occur the sensory region that maps the genitals begins to become activated. As those areas of the brain continue to stay lit up, another region called the insula begins to activate itself. The insula doesn't turn on neuronal sequences, instead it turns them off and when the insula is activated pain suppression follows which informs us of the connection between pain and pleasure. Studies have shown that women during orgasm show more resistance to pain further linking the suppression of pain impulses and orgasmic response. Women's facial expressions are indistinguishable between intense pain and intense pleasure.

With lightning speed excited responses glide from the insula to the anterior cingulate before moving on to the amygdala. The amygdala processes all kinds of intense emotional information from fear to the very pleasurable sensations of orgasm. The next area we see activity in is the hippocampus that coordinates disparate regions of the brain to act in unison. The hippocampus is involved in very strong brain activities such as seizures and there is an underlying similarity in that they both involve many regions of the brain acting together at the same time. It also has a hand in recording and playing back memories such as erotic fantasies.

After those areas have started their sequences of activation, the sequences of neuronal stimulation that began in the vagina or clitoris, moves to the prefrontal cortex an area known for behavior control, abstract thought and planning. Acting all together a triggering moment occurs when muscles begin to contract and movement becomes involuntary. Now the hypothalamus turns on and floods a woman's bloodstream with oxytocin, which is the so-called "Love hormone" giving rise to a wealth of pleasurable sensations. Oxytocin is the natural equivalent to a love potion as it encourages cuddling, bonding and loving relationships. The peak of orgasm is felt as dopamine is released and the fireworks light off in the nucleus accumbens. And then on a neurological level, the lights dim, things go quiet and peace reigns throughout the kingdom. At least until the chemicals wear off.

The amazing thing is the connections and the wiring. From stimulations occurring in the nipples, clitoris and/or vagina, electrical signals race through the body entering a tangled network in the brain that moves them through various on and off ramps like on a super highway. They in turn light up various brain regions that release chemicals triggering different responses that result in the body writhing, intense facial expressions, pleasure and peak of orgasm followed by a blissful state of consciousness. It's a ballet of choreography between body and mind that is stunning in its complexity. That it works at all is nothing short of amazing.

It also serves to underline the complexity of women's sexuality. There is no separation between a healthy body and the ability to experience sexual pleasure; they are inextricably joined together. If any single part in this chain of causation is damaged or broken, sexual response is diminished.

That is why the focus of the Menopause Plan is treating vaginal atrophy so as to maintain sexual vibrancy. When skin is damaged, nerve endings are also damaged. Without sufficient nerves to send signals to the brain the sequence of arousal, stimulation, climax and afterglow becomes broken. Libido naturally becomes suppressed as a result. Preventing this sequence from breaking down is the best goal for treating menopause. Rejuvenating already damaged tissues and restoring them to a pre-atrophy state should become the routine standard of care for women suffering the effects of menopause.

Living to 100 Years Old

Women these days are living to an average age of 81 years old, many are making it to the century mark. They will live with menopause for between thirty to forty years after it begins to assert itself and during that entire time, menopause will be changing their bodies. As we've noted some of these changes are temporary like the traditional symptoms while others creep upon a woman's body in subtle hard to detect advances that will become permanent.

What has always been missing from menopause has been a global, integrated plan for treating it. This plan needs to include education for women even before the first skipped period so they will know what's up ahead and be able to shift their thinking toward a long -term strategy for dealing with it. At pre-menopause women should consider treatments that prevent vaginal atrophy from occurring and know the best way to address the distressful symptoms like hot flashes. When menopause has established itself fully, meaning a year of no periods, the strategy will need to shift again as now the effects of menopause will move more quickly than in the earlier stages.

The most important fact that needs to be established is that menopause is a condition that once begun continues for decades and that the treatments that work best are best started early. As a woman ages the type of treatments should change, dosages adjusted and a process of adjusting then readjusting treatments begun. The end goal is clear, a woman should preserve her body so that she will age gracefully and remain sexually vibrant with lifelong vaginal health. A healthy vagina is critical to aging well, it does not matter if a woman is sexually active or not.

Why Fitness and Diet are Critical to Aging Well and Maintaining Sexual Vibrancy.

Aging well means different things to different people. We know that some women will have desire for sexual relations and others will not. There is no such thing as "Normal", normal is what is normal for the individual. That is why as one goes through life there are certain choices to be made that are right only for you. This becomes apparent when we take a look at the role of diet, nutrition, fitness, Yoga and MBSR in keeping and maintaining a healthy and vigorous body.

From a cultural perspective, we live in perilous times. There is no authoritative source that compels us to do what is best for our bodies. Most of the time it seems that quite the opposite is what occurs. Our foods are frequently full of processed materials and contain too many calories and of the wrong types. And yet that type of food is widely available, inexpensive and delicious. It encourages us to choose it, not the harder to find, more expensive natural foods that are the better choice.

We also are aware that the body does best when challenged by vigorous exercise that comes in two types, muscle building and aerobic exercise for the heart and circulation. And yet many of us spend hours lost in a digital world of friends, games, videos, shopping, Facebook and Google searches. And this doesn't count television and time spent at work or school in front of various screens and devices.

Our fast paced 21st century culture does not encourage us to make our bodies fit and healthy, it encourages us to sit in front of screens and eat. Therefore we must plan on improving things for ourselves despite the dominance of the digital and fast food worlds that increasingly pervade our lives. The combination of cultural excesses and the day-to-day difficulties of the modern world generate stress for all of us. Stress is always there sometimes forcefully asserting itself and sometimes just humming in the background.

Stress and adult life in the modern world just seem to come as a set of bookends. It is important for our health to be conscious of what makes stress arise and what will diminish its impact upon our lives. Stress kills. It's a fact. It leads to unhappiness, high blood pressure, weight gain, heart disease and even cancer. Living a healthy life means dealing effectively with stress.

Achieving a balanced life that results in decreased stress and thereby better health is a universally sought quest that is universally difficult to achieve. The Doctor' Best Advice that I offer is to be reasonable. Do not push yourself, it will likely result in failure. The best way that we know of to live a healthier life is to make small positive steps that are acceptable.

Today, maybe you will choose a healthy lunch over a fast food meal. Perhaps in the next week you will make one healthy choice of what kind of food to eat each day. Maybe you'll eat more home cooked meals and snacks. Hopefully the calories, salt and fat intake will go down. If you keep doing one small thing to eat better each day eventually you will have significantly improved your diet, nutrition and health. No soul-crushing diet regime needed, just small changes applied over time.

The same is true of fitness. Regardless of your current state of fitness improvement is possible and fairly easy to achieve. If you are currently not an active person make a conscious effort to get out and walk. Walk a block today. Maybe you'll walk two blocks tomorrow and three blocks in a few weeks. If you already have a fitness routine established, push yourself just a little harder each time you workout. No big leaps forward, just run a little faster, a little further. Swim or bike just a bit more often and so on. Bit by bit this gradualist approach can offer large-scale improvements to health. Even if you don't have the time or don't feel like it just do something positive everyday.

Diets that were once unhealthy become healthier. Fitness routines that once featured laps between the TV, refrigerator and couch now include laps around the local park. The advantage of this approach is that diets don't work very well. This is an established fact. They revolve around short-term gains and often make meals into exercises of denial. Nutrition and diet in general should be joyous and filled with delicious foods. The Mediterranean approach to food is among the world's healthiest and most delicious, if you can incorporate it's best features into your own life you will enjoy both great food and better health.

Fitness is the same but there is an additional benefit with physical action that often goes unreported. Physical action settles the mind leading to a calmer experience of life. The benefits are short term, a person must exercise daily for the benefits to be felt daily, but any increase in physical activity has an impact on the mind. Keeping weight under control is the other major benefit of fitness but there are least two others that should be talked about. Bone density and muscle mass. Part of the aging process includes the steady deterioration of bone density and muscle fiber. If too much bone density is lost, a condition called osteoporosis takes over making bones brittle and prone to fracture. Losing muscle mass makes climbing stairs and other mundane activities difficult and increases the chances of falls and injury.

Aging gracefully therefore also means being aware that bones will become weak if they are not subjected to frequent exercise. Muscles will weaken and diminish in strength if not subjected to resistance training. After many years the effects of bone and muscle loss can plainly be seen. Many older women have a stooped posture, a slowness to their walk and a fragile appearance about them. These effects of aging are both preventable and reversible but they need to be acknowledged for an effective plan counteracting these effects to be instituted.

Yoga offers women a unique approach to fitness that helps combine exercise with mind calming techniques. Additional benefits include increased flexibility and strength. For many people the best advantage of Yoga is that there are many classes available at all times of day and the group atmosphere, chance to make friends etc. can become a powerful motivator. Yoga also has been shown to help relieve menopausal symptoms, help with back pain and scoliosis. For some women it may be the correct combination of exercise, routine and group support necessary to stay with it.

Mindfulness Based Stress Reduction is a new form of mind training that draws from Buddhist meditation techniques to help focus the mind. It is widely taught in Fortune 500 companies, the military, in private seminars and universities throughout the world. Some of its advocates and teachers have become famous celebrities and offer MBSR apps such as Buddify for mobile devices and personalized training classes. As a technique of self-help it is gaining in popularity because it has been shown to help deal with stress as effectively as some medications. Women with menopausal symptoms also report that it offers relief. MBSR can be thought of as a tool to help train one's mind so as to direct it for a variety of purposes; pain relief, calming, stress reduction, insomnia and more. As an additional arrow in the quiver of weapons for taming the mind MBSR can be of benefit for living a better more healthful life.

KATHERINE

Something happened to Katherine as the estrogen treatments did their work healing the damaged tissues of her vaginal walls. She rediscovered her enjoyment of sex. Timmy turned her on, he wanted a relatively high level of sexual activity and Katherine was receptive to the concept. At 52 years old she had gone from being unable to have intercourse to it becoming an important part of her life and an important way to express her growing love for Timmy.

Katherine's appointments were scheduled at month long intervals so that we could track the changes and see if any adjustments in her medications were needed. The exam went well, the tissues were regenerating there was clearly more soft moist vaginal tissue. All the signs of a healthy vagina were present. The only thing that Katherine complained of was occasional soreness after intercourse. There was some minor irritation that I could see but from a medical standpoint there was no reason for concern.

"Soreness?" I asked, "When do you feel it, does it come and go or is it always there?" I asked getting my pen ready to make some notes.

"I'm sore after sex. During is ok but when he pulls out I feel like a scratchiness all down through there."

"Every time?" I asked.

"No, the first time we have sex its all right. By the second time it's bothering me."

"Is Timmy taking Viagra?"

"No, he just likes it twice in a row."

"Other than the irritation anything else?"

"That's it."

I put the pen down. Katherine had responded well to the vaginal estrogen that we'd been using as a topical remedy but a new issue arose. The frequency of sexual activity that she was reporting could in fact be the cause of her symptoms. The layers of vaginal tissue she'd regrown, although stronger and healthier than before, were still only a few layers thick. Over time and with other treatments there would be more tissue, more nerve endings and greater resiliency to reduce the type of irritation she was reporting. But without further treatment, her sexual experience would likely be similar to the one she was speaking about.

Katherine had achieved the ability to have pleasurable intercourse, but her vaginal walls were still not healthy enough for repeated sessions in quick succession. With some downtime between sexual relations, her vagina would have done fine with this level of treatment. The cell structures would've bounced back and become ready for another round but they needed some time between and they weren't getting it.

"Ok Katherine I have some news for you that is all good. Your vagina is much healthier than it was when we started a couple of months ago and we should continue to see steady improvement. Let's continue the ring and cream because it's working well for you. Lubrication for intercourse will help diminish the irritation and make it better feeling. But..."

Katherine looked up a little, "You said 'All good news.'"

"But there's a way to continue to improve your vaginal health which should make your experience of sex even better. There is a new FDA approved, safe and effective way to rejuvenate vaginal tissue and restore it to that of a younger woman. We've been using it with excellent results and this would be the course of treatment I might have recommended for you in about a year but since circumstances have changed which in turn have changed your needs, I'd like you to think about laser rejuvenation now. I think it's the right time and it should help you feel significant improvement without additional medication.

Katherine looked at me, "I'm listening," She said.

BETH

Beth's case of recurring vaginal and bladder infections was due to an effect of menopause that is rarely talked about. The pH level of a woman's vagina is important to maintaining the proper balance of good bacteria. As skin becomes atrophic this balance becomes upset limiting the growth of beneficial bacteria. Harmful bacteria can grow and an infection is frequently the result.

Antibiotics are effective in fighting these localized infections. But they are a temporary cure. To effectively prevent future infections from occurring it is necessary to grow the type of skin tissue that prevents the growth of harmful microorganisms and encourages the growth of beneficial ones.

The correct Menopause Plan for Beth was to first cure her bladder infection and then to return her vaginal tissue to good health. Her two prescriptions were for antibiotics and also a transdermal estrogen cream. The pills would cure the infection and the estrogen cream would begin rebuilding healthy vaginal tissue.

When Beth came in for her appointment six weeks later the infection had cleared up and she reported that she had been applying the cream as recommended.

"Great news," I said, "Feeling better?"

"Much," Beth replied, "But when do I get off the cream?"

"Let's take a look and see what we can see," I said. She headed to the exam room and I followed a few minutes later. After the physical we sat across from one another in my office.

"So? Is the cream working?" Beth asked, "I can't really tell."

"Yes, it is working I'm happy to report. In six weeks you're doing as well as we could've hoped," I said.

"Stop using the cream?" She asked.

"Not yet and maybe not for awhile. The new skin growth I see is encouraging but it needs time to heal and grow into abundant fresh tissue. The transdermal estrogen cream is a pinpoint treatment that will continue to heal the exact areas that need an estrogen boost. As this low dosage doesn't enter the bloodstream in any significant amount, it is both safe and effective to keep using it. Over time, the effects will become more noticeable and accomplish the end result we're after, an end to the vaginal and bladder infections. The pH of your vagina will stabilize at the right level so that good bacteria will be able to grow and bad bacteria will be limited."

Beth nodded at the now familiar information I was delivering. "As a result we should continue the cream and in the future we will likely lower the dosage as we continue to see improvements. For now it's working. You're happy with things so far?"

"I'm happy," Beth said. I wrote out a new prescription for her and we planned to see one another in six months unless another matter came up in the meantime.

EMMA

Emma was a 50 year-old woman who enjoyed a high level of sexual activity. She was a serial monogamist and her sexual history included affairs with both men and women. She recently met a man she was falling in love with and they'd taken it to the next level of intimacy. As a woman who had frequent sex since her teen years, her vagina was in good shape as a result. The reason for this is that with sexual arousal women experience increased blood flow to the vagina helping stabilize vaginal skin and tissue. In addition, frequent sex helps to maintain the sexual arousal circuitry that can begin to decline at anytime with decreased activity and especially during menopause's long advance.

Emma was sexually interested, easily achieved orgasms and had no sexual dysfunction whatsoever. There was no need to treat her for hot flashes, sleeplessness or irritability because she was not bothered by any of those symptoms even though they occurred from time to time. Similarly, her vagina still had an abundance of soft, moist tissue and she reported no troubling symptoms during intercourse. For Emma, the individualized treatment for menopause she required was no treatment of any kind for now. In the future, it is likely she will need some form of treatment, especially if she wishes to remain sexually active, but for now the best course of medicine is no medicine at all.

We completed her yearly physical exam and as she had no health problems and needed no prescriptions, she was good to go for another year unless the lab results kicked up something to look at more closely.

Doctors Best Advice for Emma was twofold, first a reminder about standard precautions and symptoms of STDs as she had multiple partners in the recent past. Second, was information about symptoms of menopause and vaginal atrophy that would likely occur in the future perhaps even before her next scheduled routine visit.

"Any other concerns, anything you'd like to talk about?" I asked, beginning to wrap things up.

"Actually Doctor, there is one thing."

"Sure, what?" I said putting her chart to the side.

"You know how some guys get Viagra?"

"Yes?"

"Take the little blue pill and with a little nudging they're easy to get an erection?"

"Yes?" I said.

"So, my girlfriends, their boyfriends get Viagra and they're all over them. Soon they're doing it every day, all the time. Like teenagers. So, my new guy is Brian, he's forty-one and works at Macys, very nice guy. Cute. He has a little trouble down there starting before we met. And so he goes to the doctor, gets a prescription for Viagra. And he won't take it." Emma said crossing her arms across her chest, "He doesn't want to take it."

"Does he get bad effects from it? Any side effects? Stomach issues? Headaches. Prolonged erections?"

"None."

"So why doesn't he take it?"

"You tell me?!?" Emma said.

And there I had it. Sex had become unbalanced between Emma and Brian. For whatever reasons, Brian and Emma had engines that were running at different speeds. Some people prefer sex three times a day, others want it three times a month and for others no sex at all is just fine. There is no right or wrong amount of sexual activity as long as the partners involved are both satisfied. As relative sex drives can be hard to quantify before the actual events occur, mismatches sometimes happen. In this case a mismatch of sexual balances was occurring. Viagra made it possible for Brian to match Emma's sexual pace but he wasn't interested.

"I'm thinking of spiking his beer," Emma said after we went back and forth for a minute.

"Don't do that!" I said. "Listen, all I have is general advice. Your desire for sex is stronger than his. Sometimes it goes the other way especially since they started handing out Viagra like Halloween treats to kids. For you, if your relationship can include lower sexual expectations, than you and Brian are probably going to be good together. But if this is very important to you I don't think it's realistic to think he'll want to pop a pill more often than he feels like popping a pill."

Emma looked pensive she pursed her lips together for a second, "Not the first time a guy's been almost perfect."

She turned and waved goodbye as she made her way out the door, unless there was a medical issue that arose I anticipated we'd see each other again in about a year. She was perfectly healthy and her experience of menopause seemed to be going very well.

DOCTOR'S BEST ADVICE

Doctors are always looking for something. They're like detectives searching for clues. Sometimes a clue arrives in a blood test, a lab result or a urine sample. At times clues arrive from a physical exam, a change in demeanor or a pain response when touched in a certain place. Each of these leads a doctor to either suspect or rule out illness or potential problems. As doctors make small talk with their patients they're looking for signs of breathlessness, depression, or perhaps concern about a specific topic. And they seek to follow up on all of these telltale indicators.

Most of the time they go nowhere. Sometimes they reveal a serious condition that needs to be treated.

The Doctor's Best Advice I can offer is when you are going to your annual doctor's appointment is that you prepare for it. Time with your physician will be limited unless health concerns warrant a longer visit. Patients who keep track of their health with a Symptoms Journal (More later) have a document that a doctor can review. The doctor will look for changes over time and the presence or absence of troubling symptoms. Fevers, headaches, abdominal pain, frequency of stomach problems, fatigue or sleeplessness may all be indications for a doctor to consider. The more your doctor knows the better they will be able to treat you.

At the time of the visit, it is best if you can arrive with a list of things that you'd like to ask about. Your physician can answer all your questions, review your medications and note any changes that have occurred since the last appointment.

The doctor will be similarly prepared. There is a guideline that underlies your visit and it's called the Interval Medical History. It is a basic way for a doctor to gather information for the purpose of diagnosis and treatment and to enter it into a file for future review or reference. In addition to that part of the annual appointment there will also be a blood pressure test, sometimes having blood drawn as appropriate and a urine sample collected usually by a medical technician or physician's assistant. The doctor will conduct the physical exam. Then a conversation will typically take place where the doctor reviews the findings and asks if there are any other concerns the patient may have. In conclusion, the results will come back within two weeks and be reviewed. Any results that indicate further testing, referrals or additional office visits are needed will be done at that time.

What doctors are doing in an exam is evaluating a patient's overall health and their needs going forward. Doctor's questions roam from personal habits to family history and past medical events. Each question may in turn lead to additional questions as the physician seeks to include or rule out the need for further inquiry or perhaps testing.

Most doctors ask questions like these as they take a patient's history. "Are there any changes to your health since your last visit?"

"How are things at home, any unusual stress?"

"Are you taking any medications including herbals, recreational drugs, alcohol or cigarettes?"

"Are you sexually active? If so, how many partners and are they men, women or both?"

"Do you have any discomfort with sex? Pain? Burning? Itching? Odor? Discharge?"

"If you have pain is it more in the vagina or the abdomen or both?"

"Any pain when you urinate? Bowel movements? Do you ever see any blood?"

"Are there any tests you think we should do? STD's? Any questions about cancer screening?"

"When was your last period? Any problems? Is it heavy or painful?

"Any questions about contraception or family planning?"

"Any significant changes in family health? Cancer? Diabetes? Stroke? Heart disease?"

At each of these questions there might be a reply that opens up the door to a flurry of additional follow-ups coupled with blood tests, MRI's, X-Rays, ultrasound or many other diagnostic tools at our disposal. The reason I am a big fan of patients keeping a Symptoms Journal is that by having a window into a woman's health, patterns over an extended period of time can become apparent. Making it less likely to need to order diagnostic tests as the clues may be picked up more easily. Secondly it will help us pinpoint what tests are most appropriate to do first thereby limiting tests that might have been avoided if more information was available.

TRACEY

The technicians at Radiology were finished with me. The CAT machine was tabulating its results and soon via the hospital's interconnected data network it would be whisked down to the physician who was evaluating my case.

The ride back to the Emergency Room was a repeat of the same parade of overhead fluorescent lights except in reverse. By the time they wheeled me back downstairs I was starting to feel a little better and it wasn't just from the medications they'd injected me with. I was starting to come around. I sat up a little and talked to my husband. By now the Emergency Room had filled up with new arrivals and there was no longer a place for me in a curtained off vestibule. I was parked between two other people who were also awaiting results.

As new patients arrived by ambulance or as walk-ins, there would be a flurry of activity as doctors, nurses and technicians schooled around them like white-coated fish. Once evaluated, medicated and priority care dispensed, one by one they were all sent separate ways through the hospital corridors. One went to Pediatrics, another got sent to the 6th floor Obstetrics ward, still another journeyed onward to Urology.

A woman came in by ambulance confused as to why she was in the Emergency Room and not at another hospital where her doctor had an appointment with her which seemed to confuse everyone else as to why she was here at all. My husband handed me some water to drink and I leaned back and slept for a few minutes.

"Tracey?" A soft voice said and I opened my eyes to see Jennifer an old friend and the new ER Doc on call. She'd come in while I was in Radiology, "We got the results." She swiveled a computer monitor around and showed me the output from the CAT scan. She didn't say anything assuming I would read the scan and leap to the proper conclusion because it was so obvious. All I could make out were blurry lines. An awkward moment passed.

"It's a kidney stone," She said at last.

And I was both relieved and flummoxed. Normally kidney stones pass by themselves causing a lot of pain and distress but they're gone within a few days. My kidney stone got hung up and wasn't passing, throwing my whole system into critical distress.

As a doctor I now realized I should have recognized the symptoms of my growing health emergency sooner but I chose to ignore them. For two weeks prior to my falling unconscious and going into shock, I had lower back pain and stomach trouble but I powered through. As a young medical intern it had been drummed into me that any minor illness was to be downplayed because the work of medicine had to continue. A doctor simply wasn't allowed to cancel office hours, surgeries or delivering babies just because of an upset stomach or muscle soreness. This ethic of devoted work at all costs had served me just fine for over twenty-five years. Right up until the day it didn't.

Now I had become a victim of my own overwork. Too busy to pay attention to my own health, my health was now paying attention to me. Big time. I was in severe pain and could barely walk. The stone had not passed and there was a chance I could pass out from the pain again. Jennifer gave me a handful of prescriptions and my husband and I slowly and painfully made it home.

After a few days I felt better and returned to the office. Janet, my best friend and colleague took over my deliveries. Days passed in a kind of haze of ill health and after about two weeks I finally passed the stone that almost killed me. I returned to a less hectic version of my earlier routine as my body continued to heal and prepared to pass what would turn out to be a few additional mineral accretions as they are sometimes called. For the next year I was exhausted, couldn't eat and felt sick almost every day.

Patients who hadn't seen me in awhile commented favorably on how thin I looked. I would smile and nod appreciatively at the compliment as it was of course, well intended. But I had lost twenty pounds and had grown considerably weaker over the year. It wasn't that I didn't want to eat, it's that everything I tried to eat repulsed me and gave me a stomachache. For the first time since I was nineteen years old and had decided to pursue a career in medicine, I realized that I might have to quit. I could no longer keep up.

SOFIA

Sofia and I had been seeing one another every six months for routine follow-ups. So when she came in for her regular appointment we said hello and made small talk for a few minutes. She noted that I had lost weight since she'd seen me last and I said "'Yes I've lost a little weight recently.'"

We quickly went through the Interval Medical History and when I asked, "Are you sexually active?" She replied that she was. That was a change since six months ago.

"Are you seeing men, women or both and how many?"

"One man."

"How long has it been since your last period?"

"A year."

"Any questions about birth control? Menopause? STD's?"

Sofia shook her head no.

"Any medical issues you'd like to bring up, things you'd like to talk about?" Sofia looked at her toes for a few seconds and then our eyes met.

"There is one thing that's come up," She began, "Sex…" She trailed off, "Is not like how I remember."

"Can you tell me what you're feeling? Why it seems different?"

"It seems…" Sofia said, "Not as intense as I remember it. It's more like the same actions but without the same pleasure."

"Are you able to have orgasms?" I asked.

She had to find the right words and it took her a few seconds, "After a lot of stimulation. Penetration doesn't do it for me. Oral I'm better, but it's…different."

We had already completed the physical exam and I could see her vaginal tissue had become drier and thinner in just the past six months. If Sofia had been receptive to topical hormone treatment earlier, we could have prevented the condition from asserting itself. I asked about her choices regarding lubrication and found her to be informed about what to use and when.

Sofia's complaint was the result of vaginal atrophy and although using a lubricant could ease the mechanics of intercourse, it did less to improve the blood flow that is critical to achieving sexual arousal. Also there was still the issue of the wiring of the sex organs response to her brain. These connections had grown weaker and their ability to generate a signal to the brain had lessened. Therefore the sexual response had weakened. The embodiment of this change was Sofia's sexual responsiveness had diminished to a noticeable degree. If she did not have a new man in her life or if sexual activity was not important to her, this may not have become an issue. Circumstances being what they were however, a new love relationship had created a new sexual need and her body was not responding in the way she expected or desired.

We spoke of earlier conversations about estrogen and the changes in vaginal health that occurs when it declines. She remembered the science behind the changes in her body and we both restated her preference for organic treatments. For Sofia, the possibilities of medical treatment via Hormone Replacement Therapy were unacceptable. She had a strong aversion to hormones and I noted that she had done her research. Sofia pulled out a thick printout of reasons why women should avoid Hormone Replacement Therapy at all costs and handed it to me. She spoke to me of her concerns about breast cancer, stroke and heart disease all attributable, she told me to HRT. When Sofia handed me the printout, I needed to look no further. She had Googled Hormone Replacement Therapy and been guided to the Women's Health Initiative's report from 2002.

The WHI's report was widely covered in the media with headlines that outlined the increased breast cancer risk as a result of Hormone Replacement Therapy. Overnight, prescriptions for HRT plummeted as physicians immediately avoided prescribing them and patients expressed outright fear of taking them.

I assured Sofia that I knew the study very well. I understood what the WHI studied was not what we do now to treat menopause. Those were treatments of a past day when every woman was going to be "Cured" of her menopause by relentless doses of estrogen. Today the treatments are targeted, do not last for long periods of time and use lower doses that are safe and effective. Application of estrogen may include systemic oral or transdermal bio-identical or synthetic agents with dosing options that can be optimized for the individual woman's symptoms and adjusted according to her response. Vaginal treatments with estrogen tablets, rings or cream use minimal doses locally and are barely detectable in the bloodstream.

Today's state-of-the-art treatment for women undergoing meno-pause is an individualized plan that treats their temporary symptoms as well as preventing and/or treating vaginal atrophy. This is a new way to treat menopause and it is widely used by women doctors to treat their own menopause. This is true of myself as well as many of my friends and colleagues. Not only wouldn't I put myself at risk, I would never put a patient at risk.

With Sofia's case the options for treating her growing sexual dysfunc-tion were limited. Her aversion to certain kinds of medications made laser rejuvenation the best treatment for her. Had she remained sexu-ally inactive or wished to begin low dose hormone therapy the course of action would have been different. The medications if given time to work, would have improved her vaginal atrophy, and she could have resumed sexual activity with improvement in her vaginal symptoms.

After a period of time her medications would be adjusted and as she progressed through her menopause we would fine-tune them. But in keeping true to Sofia's preferences, we needed another Plan.

"Ok," I said as I put my pen down and closed her file. "There are two things I want to discuss with you in depth about where you are right now, what may be the best choices to make going forward and what alternatives we have to treat your condition. The first thing we need to talk about is the Women's Health Initiative of 2002 what it said, what it doesn't say and why you shouldn't be scared of hormones. I'm not trying to change your mind, it's just that I'd like you to hear the facts from a physician-scientist who has treated thousands of women, knows all the data, went through menopause herself and wants only the best for you. The second thing we need to talk about, and this is especially important if you decide that you want to avoid hormones is the Mona Lisa Touch."

Sofia looked at me with a curious smile, "Mona Lisa? Like in Leonardo da Vinci?"

"No," I said. "That's why we need to talk."

CHAPTER 3

TREATING MENOPAUSE EFFECTIVELY

MANY WOMEN ARE frightened of hormones and do not wish to consider using them. Their fear is misplaced. Today, the treatments available are safe and effective and can provide benefits that far exceed the slight risks to women who use them. I have used them myself as do many other women obstetrician-gynecologists to treat their menopause.

The place where the fear started was in a study that began in the 1990's that found an increase in the rates of breast cancer among women who had used a medication called Prempro* that was once widely pre-scribed as a "Cure-All" for menopause. It was the wrong combination of hormones to use and it is now not commonly used in that manner or for that purpose. At the time it was prescribed the science of meno-pause was in its infancy and what science existed, was dominated by men. Their concept of treatment was not consistent with the treatment even young women doctors of the same era were likely to prescribe.

The research project was called the Women's Health Initiative and it was a massive study that began in the 1990's to track 160,000 women over eight years. It had a sharp focus. The study was designed to find out if Hormone Replacement Therapy in the form of Prempro would lower the risk of heart disease in menopausal women between 50-79 years old. Scientists had long known that women had a lower risk for heart disease than men of the same age but that changed at menopause when their risk went up. Everyone wanted to find out why.

---

* *Prempro is a single pill which combines a fixed dose of both synthetic progesterone and estrogen. It is highly effective at treating symptoms of menopause like hot flashes without causing bleeding in women with a uterus*

From the same datasets scientists would also be able to draw out important information about cancer rates, strokes, osteoporosis and other illnesses. The headlines that blared around the world heralded the fact that researchers had found a significant increase in breast cancer among the 160,000 women who had taken part in the study. In 2002 the study was discontinued.

This finding was true as far as it went and events over the past fifteen years highlight the complexities of what they found. The most important fact is that 160,000 women were given the same drug to use for extended periods of time, many had been using it for eight or nine years. The second relevant fact for women today is that there was no individualization of care. The thinking was that estrogen fixes menopause.

As a physician looking for facts that will drive the decisions I'll be making for myself, my family, friends and patients what I found was encouraging not alarming. Even though we no longer prescribe those medications nor use them in the way the researchers studied, there were still interesting things to look at. Colon-rectal cancers in the same group went down by 27%. Osteoporosis rates declined. Menopause symptoms were eased to such an extent for so many women they preferred to stay on their HRT regime. There were also findings that went to the core of their initial research and they found that Prempro did not help prevent heart disease or strokes in women.

As far as breast cancer rate increases? They were statistically significant for users of Prempro but they could not make a direct case that Prempro causes cancer. It's a confusing result but essentially what they're explaining to us is that across a pool of 160,000 women significantly more than the expected number of breast cancers were reported. However, to tie a single case of cancer to a specific woman who used Prempro became very hard to establish.

Cancer has so many causations that it is nearly impossible to find a direct link. There can be family history that tends toward cancer it could have come from environmental factors or even certain foods. Medications may have been a causal factor but there may have been a dozen others. As various cases wound their way through the courts as breast cancer victims made their case that Prempro was the cause of their illness, the link was almost impossible to prove.

According to Wikipedia over 13,000 cases were brought and out of the class action suits and individual lawsuits only one case was found for the plaintiff. So, the answer is, did Prempro cause a rise in breast cancer? The answer is maybe. That's why it is no longer used in the manner studied by the Women's Health Initiative. "Maybe" is not acceptable.

The Women's Health Initiative had an interesting section all the way near the bottom under a heading called "Limitations". In this section they state that they did not study low dosage hormone therapies and transdermal application methods. They did note that the ring and cream approach that is currently in use held promise as a treatment for vaginal atrophy as its effects mimicked the naturally occurring process. This local application coupled with individualized treatment uses such low dosages as to be absorbed only by the surrounding tissue and is barely detectable in the bloodstream.

In the past fifteen years since the WHI released its report, this small aside near the bottom under the heading "Limitations" has become the best way to treat the symptoms of menopause. Until 2015 there was really no alternative to treating vaginal atrophy except by reintroducing estrogen to a woman's body to replace what could no longer be generated naturally. Vaginal estrogen remained the best treatment for the majority of women.

Then something new appeared on the horizon.

It was new in the sense that it had become available for the treatment of vaginal atrophy but really it had been around for many years used for a different application. This was the device plus software package that has become known as the "Mona Lisa Touch". It was new to the world of gynecology but not to the world of plastic surgery. The Mona Lisa Touch uses the same fractional ablation laser technology that millions of men and women have used for skin rejuvenation as a non-surgical facelift.

As a plastic surgery tool it has been around for many years effectively treating skin that had become dry, wrinkled and aged. The basic concept behind it is that the laser zaps the skin cells exciting new skin growth to occur. The new skin is noticeably fresher, tauter and healthier and that is why it's been a favorite of everyone from Hollywood movie stars to schoolteachers. It works very well for the purpose it was intended to serve.

After a rigorous testing period the FDA approved the vaginal rejuvenation laser for use in gynecologic applications. The high technology Italian company that perfected the treatment parameters for the vaginal laser application also invented a specialized hand tool to make it work as a package for vaginal rejuvenation that is efficient and safe. The unique aspect of the Mona Lisa Touch system however is the software package that allows the laser to be used in a pinpoint manner guided zap by zap by a trained doctor. In addition, the intensity of the laser can be micro-adjusted for individualized care.

The Mona Lisa Touch has been available in Europe for many years but the licensing process delayed its introduction in the USA until recently. It is still not well known to either physicians or patients but as they are introduced to the evidence of its results, more women will be able to benefit from this important new treatment option. It is exciting for doctors to have a safe and effective non-hormonal treatment available for women experiencing vaginal atrophy caused by menopause.

The medical trials for the device were conducted at the Cleveland Clinic and it proved the rarest of all medical innovations. It became an instant hit. This breakthrough restored sexual functioning in women who had lost it. This was a new way to treat vaginal atrophy helping restore a woman's vagina to a state similar to that of a younger woman.

Just like with facial rejuvenation treatments by zapping the effected areas, new growth is excited to grow in a similar manner that estrogen once excited new tissue to grow. The doctor has a specific order to follow as the treatment progresses through the vagina with computer assisted guidance linked to the laser. It is a less than fifteen-minute procedure that is done in-office with no anesthesia needed and no downtime.

Sexual activity can resume in about a week. The only after effect that is typical is a kind of scratchy feeling that goes away after a few days. Some women experience a discharge or slight spotting. There is no pain during or as a result of the treatment.

Maximum results are achieved after three sessions six weeks apart. Each session requires the doctor to change the settings on the laser-software package to achieve the optimum treatment levels. At the completion of treatment a woman's vagina will be rejuvenated. Symptoms usually continue to gradually improve for up to six months as the tissues respond to the treatments. There will be an increase in soft, moist vaginal tissue, dryness will diminish and in its place will be a vagina that is much healthier.

Many women obstetrician-gynecologists have been treated with this method including myself. The Mona Lisa Touch yields excellent results and in the years to come, as its success is better known, it will become a widely used treatment for vaginal atrophy. At this time, the treatment is brand new and there are few Mona Lisa Touch machines available and very few trained doctors. In the next few years we are predicting that for the correct patients, this will be a common treatment for vaginal atrophy. There simply is no other safe, effective alternative that works this well without hormones or other medications.

ASK THE DOCTOR
QUESTIONS & ANSWERS

The Menopause Plan focuses on education and information to help guide women to make correct choices for themselves. By being informed of what menopause is, what age it can begin, learning about one's family history and so on, a woman is able to prepare herself for tomorrow's health needs.

The science behind menopause, estrogen levels, hormone balancing, transdermal patches and all of that is not what is most important. The important thing for women to be aware of is that menopause changes over time with different symptoms coming and going. Staying healthy, regardless of being sexually active or not requires ongoing treatment beginning with the first skipped period and continuing into old age.

Q: *"Doctor Fein I understand the laser thing, but why don't you use that in the beginning of menopause?"*

A: "As menopause begins vaginal atrophy is minimal. It needs to be followed as it is progressive but it moves slowly in most women. Also its effect on sexual activity is usually gradual and subtle and it may take many years of menopause before it becomes a problem. What we try and do is to treat the vagina as it begins its descent into atrophy so as to forestall the worst effects. For younger women mild medications are very effective, when a woman gets older the same medications may not have the same benefits. We can change the medicines, we can change how they are delivered to the effected tissue but the fact is that vaginal atrophy is progressive.

At a certain point, the medicines don't work as well as they once did or perhaps the woman using them started using them later in life than would have been optimal. At this point vaginal rejuvenation becomes the best treatment. It's not the first line of defense but when it's the right time to use it, it works really well."

Q: *"Doctor Fein my mother had breast cancer how does that effect what kind of medicines I should take?"*

A: "That's an excellent question. Breast cancer in the family increases the risks of breast cancer for the kids too and so we need to be cautious. Vaginal estrogen, the ring and cream will be fine as they don't work their way into the bloodstream in any quantity that will increase risk. Controlling the amount of estrogen you are exposed to is very important in any treatment and its important you mention your family history to your doctor. Should a real need develop however, it is possible to use systemic medications in low dosages for short durations. Finding the right treatment that is both effective and safe is the highest priority."

Q: *"What was your most challenging menopause case?"*

A: "That would be Clara. Clara was a sixty three year old patient of mine who had so many medical problems that treating her gynecologic issues was really the least of it. She had a heart condition and diabetes; bad knees, a bad back and she weighed nearly three hundred pounds on a five foot five frame. Her skin was in terrible shape and the diabetes only exacerbated the situation. Her vaginal health was bad. The skin was atrophied and prone to infections and she had gotten both vaginal and bladder infections in the past few years and her suffering was immense.

"It was hard to see how she'd have any comfortable position to sit, stand or lie down as the outer part of her vagina was inflamed and so painful to the touch it was difficult to conduct an exam. The diabetes made all skin issues very important so my care of her was ongoing and I tried to make her feel better in any way I could. Whenever she was in my office I felt so sad because the woman was living in a world of pain and there was so little I could really do for her. Getting better for her really meant getting her blood sugar levels under control and that's best managed by a diabetic specialist. In the absence of an improvement in her diabetes it was hard to forecast a really positive outcome."

Q: *"Can you talk a little but about STD's?"*

A: "Absolutely, this is an important topic. Many women complain that men over a certain age are reluctant to use condoms. This could potentially expose women to a wide variety of problems. Also the most common sexually transmitted infections gynecologists see are viral conditions like Genital Herpes and HPV or Human Papilloma

Virus. Both are difficult to detect so many people affected don't know they have them and that of course, makes it more likely they'll pass them on to others. As always, prevention is better than a cure. Talk to your partner and be completely honest about yourself and your past. The more you're open and speak honestly the easier it'll be for him or her to share. This is best done well before the moment becomes heated when let's face it, holding back becomes way more difficult.

"And unfortunately once in a while STD testing is imperfect, it gives a false negative or a false positive and retesting becomes necessary. So knowing your partner has recently been tested is really not 100% foolproof protection, there's no guarantee. This is why it is best to reserve physical relationships to people you can trust with your future health."

Q: *"What are the symptoms of menopause?"*

A: Menopause is by definition when a woman does not have a period for 12 months. When women ask me what symptoms I should expect as I get close to menopause age I tell them that the symptoms can be highly variable. There are the traditional ones; loss of libido, skipped periods, hot flashes, insomnia and mood swings. But they can come and go unpredictably and not all women even experience one of them let alone all of them. Many women begin to have increasing changes in their periods with them getting shorter and lighter but also closer together. Some women just stop having periods. A woman can expect her periods to become increasingly less predictable starting in her forties. About a third of women suffer severe symptoms that they find disrupt their lives and these can be treated. See your doctor. Keep a Symptoms Journal so it is clear what is most troubling and to help initiate a treatment plan and also monitor how well it's working

THE SYMPTOMS JOURNAL & DOCTOR'S APPOINTMENT

Keeping track of your health should begin as early as possible through the use of a notebook, diary or journal. Mobile devices are not the best because at a certain point you will want to show this to a doctor and its better for them if you can just open a page in a notebook with the correct dates, hand it to them and begin your discussion from there. Scrolling through data on a small screen can be difficult and may take up valuable time better spent on more important matters.

The information your doctor will be interested in includes how many days do you bleed or spot, when is it heavy or light? Do you have abdominal pain? How often? Is it in relation to meals or certain foods? Is it in the stomach or vaginal areas? Are you coughing or having trouble breathing? Any health related issue deserves a quick note along with the date. Your physician will be scanning the information for important changes that may have occurred over time that can help diagnose or perhaps treat you better.

Getting the most out of your doctor's appointment assumes that a patient arrives prepared. Bring the Symptoms Journal and a plastic bag with all the medications and supplements you're taking so that they can be screened for any dangers or interactions. Let the doctor know right up front about any health changes, concerns or family illnesses since your last visit. Update your file with the correct health insurance contact and email info so that phone calls and lab results can be conveyed quickly.

Doctor's visits, especially if you have disturbing symptoms can be very stressful. It's true for all patients and its also true for when doctors become patients. They're not crazy about it either when it's their turn to be on the other end of the speculum or stethoscope. The best advice for both doctors who become patients and patients who are going to the doctor's office is to try and relax. Your doctor is your ally in good health. It's good to be prepared with your Symptoms Journal and baggie full of meds but it's better to be calm and ready to work with your doctor to help make you as healthy as you can be.

MADELINE

Madeline's next visit wasn't for over six months. I hadn't heard from her and in the doctor world that's good news. If a patient is being bothered by illness or symptoms you expect to hear from them promptly. She popped in wearing a pair of diamond and gold earrings paired with a matching necklace and a big smile. She appeared to be a happy woman of 47 years.

"Where'd you last leave me?" Madeline asked.

"Mood swings were the main issue," I said recalling our last visit while simultaneously flipping through her folder, "Complicated by a uterine fibroid."

"No," Madeline said.

"And we gave you an SSRI."

"Yes and no."

"Ok, what?" I said looking at her.

"You last left me at the conniving girl curator who seduced my Chagall from Murray. Does that jog your memory?"

"I do remember. When you last left I was torn between feeling sorry for you and concerned you might murder Murray. How'd it turn out?"

"Murray is pathetic around twenty five year old women but he bought me a Warhol to compensate."

"Really, which one?" I asked.

"Elvis."

"No!"

"Yes. So he made up for it but I now forbid him from being alone with younger women who work for museums. He must always be escorted."

"And he's good with that?"

"I pointed out that we don't have a pre-nup and that I can take my hundred million and go anyplace I damn well please. So yes, on balance I'd have to say he's good with it."

"Well played," I said.

"So now, I assume you want me up in the stirrups?"

"Yes," I replied as she climbed onto the exam table.

"Fine, let's get on with it. Has anyone ever told you how undignified this entire thing is?" Madeline asked peering between her spread legs and upturned feet.

"No actually you're the first," I said as I inserted the speculum into her vagina.

After Madeline had dressed we sat down in my office. I wrote out a new prescription and we talked for a few moments.

"Any changes in my meds?" She asked.

"Very little change from last time. The SSRI is helping with the mood swings, yes?"

"Yeah, I think it's doing its job."

"The fibroids are about the same. You said you had very little bleeding?"

"Infrequent and not much."

"How's your sex life?"

"Twice a month like clockwork."

"Any irritation? Soreness? Difficulty with intercourse, any pain?"

"No, it's as thrilling as ever."

"Is Murray taking Viagra?"

"No I've forbidden it. Twice a month is perfect and he seems capable of that amount of sexual ferocity."

I nodded in acknowledgment, "So let's recap. The SSRI is working for your mood swings and hot flashes?" Madeline nodded yes. "The fibroids aren't causing a ruckus so its better to leave them alone, menopause will eventually lessen the symptoms. We won't be using estrogen for the vaginal atrophy because it will worsen the fibroids plus you aren't having any sexual difficulties so there's no urgency. I'd say you're good to go until next time or if something else comes up. Your Menopause Plan seems like its working well. Anything else you can think of?"

Madeline didn't have anything else for us to go over so we said our goodbyes for another six months.

HANNAH

The next time I saw Hannah she was playing a Mom who murdered her brother in a bizarre insurance murder-for-hire plot on Law and Order. She looked great and I made a mental note to tell her when she came in for an appointment that I enjoyed her creep-me-out performance.

Eventually appointment day rolled around and after I told her about my appreciation for her acting she told me about her husband, vagina and libido issues. Where we last left it she would try to reinvigorate the sexy side of her life through romance and we'd try to reinvigorate her private parts with vaginal estrogen. I was eager to hear both parts of the update.

"Did the Tantric thing," Hannah said referring to an Eastern sexual practice.

"Really? How'd you find a guru?" I asked.

"Craig's List," Hannah said, "He's a Tibetan lama actually, Stanley calls him a 'Renegade monk,' he's got a practice in the West 30's where he teaches couples how to, shall we say, have very long lasting sexual relations with a big impact at the end."

"Is he in the room with you?" I asked a bit unclear on how these things work.

"No!" Hannah replied, "He's NOT in the room. He teaches you stuff then you go home and practice it all on your own, then you meet again and talk about the experience."

"How's it work out?"

"The marriage is improved."

As Hannah's appointment progressed we went through the battery of questions that might reveal something deeper going on beneath the surface and there were no indications of ill health. After the physical exam, it was clear that her initial difficulties with vaginal atrophy had improved. There was a substantial improvement, "How's your sexual vibrancy?"

"I'm in a good place," Hannah said.

"Medications, from what I've seen are working fine?" I asked.

"I'm happy. I see results."

"Want to stick with what we got?" I offered.

"I think so. The Estring and the cream are working pretty well, I don't mind using them, I can keep to the routine."

"Then we have a Plan." I said closing the folder.

"We have a Plan." Hannah agreed.

That was the small triumph for a physician specialist working in a small field; Hannah had a Menopause Plan. One of the most interesting facets of practicing medicine is witnessing patients and friends over long periods of time and how they change. Some of my patients come to me for a first visit in their seventies while others come to me in their forties. Regardless of age it is a physician's role to teach as well as to prescribe and diagnose and teaching is something that is woven deeply into the fabric of medicine. Patients need to be informed of what is happening with their bodies, what the future holds and what the most beneficial treatments for them might be. In the case of menopause, the more information a woman has and the earlier she receives it, the better her experience of menopause is likely to be.

The important point is that there are as many Menopause Plans as there are women. Some begin menopause at forty years old and have more severe symptoms both initially and in years to come. Others have barely any symptoms at all and their vaginal atrophy is greatly delayed over an average woman's experience. Many women are happy with Hormone Replacement Therapies and others want something more organic or natural. The medications and treatments that every woman receives should be consistent with her values, life and personal expectations. These are all elements that provide the foundation for a successful Menopause Plan.

Sex in all its variations, is an excellent example of this. Women enjoy sex in greater or lesser amounts depending on their personal tastes, pleasure in having sex, orgasmic capability, stress load, overall health, vaginal health, family and career. Too much stress and even a sexually interested woman will likely not be in the mood.

The impact of this for generating a Menopause Plan is that sex matters. If sex is not a regular activity, there may never be a need for treating vaginal atrophy beyond transdermal low dose estrogen rings and/or creams. If sexual activity is more often, prolonged or intense than a different plan should be formulated which may include laser rejuvenation at an earlier age.

The Menopause Plan that is right for one woman will not be the best plan for another woman. Age when menopause began, family history, personal preferences and whether or not a woman is sexually active all need to be considered. By having a Menopause Plan the most harmful effects of menopause can be avoided and the best overall health achieved.

BETH

Beth continued the therapy as we discussed for a full year and when I did an examination after a year of treatment, both she and I were pleased at the results.

"How are you feeling?" I asked, "A solid year and no infections."

"Thank gosh." Beth said.

"I'm happy to tell you that from what I saw in the physical exam your vagina is in much better health. The skin is now full of bumps and folds, its not taut and inelastic like it was a year ago. This is a sign of good healthy skin and that in turns means the pH balance will be improved, the bad bacteria will diminish and the chances of getting another infection go way down."

"Alright!" Beth said at the news.

"Let's reduce the dosage to one time a week, stay with that and we'll do another checkup in six months. If there're no other issues I think you're good to go. But let's talk about one last thing."

"Sure Doc." Beth said.

"Sex."

"Oh Lord."

"I know that you're not currently sexually active but if you start dating again and wish to have sexual intercourse we'll need to change your Menopause Plan."

"Hmmm. Ok. Why?"

"Your vaginal health is now good enough to prevent the conditions that give rise to bladder or vaginal infections, but the tissue is not healthy enough for sexual activity. If you begin a sexual relationship we'll need to move to laser rejuvenation, the Mona Lisa Touch. But at this point there's no need. We've reached a good balance between your lifestyle and the stage of menopause you're in. Things are balanced and we should continue to have success with the transdermal cream alone. But tell me if sex becomes an issue and then we'll make an adjustment? Ok?" I asked.

"Ok," Beth said. She continued to come in for regular checkups and other than a few minor issues her course of treatment has been the same for over five years now. The tissue of her vagina is now much healthier using the cream alone and she hasn't had a bladder or vaginal infection since.

TRACEY

My individual path to a Menopause Plan for myself was more circuitous than for most of my patients. After I stumbled home from the Emergency

Room I was hoping that the episode was behind me and that soon I would pass the stone. And eventually I did, I slowly got back to work delivering babies, seeing patients and reviewing lab results. The schedule was always packed and I raced from here to there. The problem was I still felt sick.

Food was a problem, it just didn't appeal to me. I lost over twenty pounds and became deeply fatigued. My mood was in the basement and my stomach was always upset. Over the next year I passed six more stones and when I went to my urologist for a check-up she got very serious with me very fast.

"Any blood?" She asked.

"Yes but it's from the stones passing through, just damaged the tissues."

"Dr. Tracey? You're diagnosing yourself, please stop. How often and how much? When did it first appear?" Sandy went on for a few minutes with an increasingly worried look on her face as she furiously scribbled notes in my folder. "Here's what we need to do, CAT scan, cystoscopy, X-Ray, sonogram and a Gyn exam right away. Not tomorrow, today."

"Cancer?" I said my voice suddenly very small.

"Maybe. We'll find out." Sandy said.

What followed was not the blur of events many people describe. Rather it was a series of events in sharp relief. As a doctor, I knew very well what she was hunting for. I had presented myself as a patient with a kidney problem that did not resolve the way these things normally resolve. Sandy had seen what I was in denial about; fatigue, bleeding, loss of appetite, weight loss. The correct thing to rule in or out as a diagnosis, was uterine, bladder or kidney cancer. Those were the illnesses that best suited my symptoms.

In fast succession I went through a second CAT scan, a cystoscopy, sonogram and an X-Ray. Sandy's possible diagnosis made a hidden emotional part of me rise to the surface and coping with a normally stressful life just got exponentially more difficult. I became totally exhausted and just wanted to sleep.

The next thing I needed to do was see my gynecologist that would be the next day at three. In the meantime the results started to come in. The X-Ray was inconclusive and the cystoscopy results were negative. But the CAT scan results were saying possible metastatic uterine cancer. I was a wreck. It didn't matter what my doctors told me in consoling terms, I knew what these results meant. I had reviewed similar findings with many women over the years. And as I lay there exhausted waiting for the next turn of the wheel, I faded into a dreamless sleep.

The next day was bright without a cloud in the sky. I sat and drank coffee with my husband and we waited together until three. At Janet's office we sat and talked for a few minutes until it grew pointless. It was time for the exam. The physical exam in a case like this is a large determining factor in both diagnosis and treatment. The CAT scan, sonogram and cystoscopy can reveal false positives in addition to accurately diagnosing real illnesses. But when a physical exam is conducted and the actual tissues looked at by a specialist, many things can be proven or ruled out that are impossible by imaging technologies alone.

I peered between my spread legs and upturned feet and said to Janet who was just beginning to insert the speculum, "Has anyone ever told you how undignified this whole thing is?"

Janet looked up at me sharply and repeated the line we've both said a thousand times, "No, actually you're the first. Now shut up I'm working." Which made us both smile, as her harsh reply was something neither of us would say to a patient but between doctors it was amusing.

I tried not to squirm but the speculum was uncomfortable. Janet took a very long time and I was thinking that if I was a patient I might write a bad review on the web because she was taking so long and I HAD TO KNOW NOW!

After an eternity she gestured that she was done. I took my feet from the stirrups and swung my legs over the side of the exam table. She patted me on the shoulder and looked into my eyes.

"The CAT scan was wrong or they read it wrong. You do not have uterine cancer. But I do have some news that you need to hear."

I looked up at her, in an instant my heart was freed from the fear of cancer and in another moment concern welled inside of me again. I searched her face for a long moment before she spoke.

"Your vaginal atrophy is getting pretty advanced and we need to start treating it with an estrogen ring and some cream," She started to write out a prescription. And I started laughing and crying in the same moment. The strong emotions that doctors train to keep under guard all came surging out. My husband hugged me.

"You're going to be all right." Janet said as she handed me two prescriptions, "Now get out of here I have sick patients to see."

SOFIA

The most troubling problem that Sofia's menopause presented was that sex had become much less pleasurable due to vaginal dryness. Her condition was due to the fact that her menopause started early. Because of early onset of menopause the vaginal issues she was experiencing were of the type frequently seen in older women. Sofia had elected to avoid hormone therapy in favor of herbal and natural treatments and that direction had proven effective for her. Until now.

At this point in Sofia's menopause a new element had introduced itself into her Menopause Plan; she had a lover. And that changed the dynamic of her treatment. We had two elements converging. One was the early onset of menopause with accompanying untreated vaginal atrophy and secondly the desire for heightened sexual activity.

A dry vagina makes for bad sex. Vaginal atrophy creates dryness, thinness of tissues, difficulty producing natural lubrication, difficulty in achieving orgasm and in more advanced cases painful or impossible vaginal intercourse. We have seen that vaginal atrophy can begin even before the first skipped period and continues until the most senior of years. It can be the worst effect of menopause and if left untreated, it is both progressive and permanent.

Preventing vaginal atrophy means preventing sexual dysfunction from occurring in the first place. The Menopause Plan says that women shouldn't wait until they can't have sex, experience bad sex or have problems getting to an orgasm. These conditions, from a physician's point of view, should never have arisen. They should have been prevented through an active program of treatment that begins with the start of menopause and continues for decades to come. Menopause for most women will begin around age fifty and can continue for another thirty to forty years. In that entire span of time, estrogen will be depleted from their bodies and their vaginal tissues will suffer as a result. This can be prevented by early and proper treatment that is individualized for each and every woman. No two women are alike and no two women have identical experiences of menopause. That is why every woman needs a Menopause Plan.

That is why Sofia and I sat face to face and discussed what to do next.

"Let's talk philosophy," I began.

"Mine is no hormones," Sofia said.

"I know, that's not what I'm getting at," I replied, "What I was going to say was that we all make choices. We either do something in the here and now or else we live with the existing conditions. In the case of vaginal atrophy, it's not like diabetes where if you don't take insulin, you'll die. We're talking sex here, it's very personal as to how important it is to any individual but it's not life or death. It's more quality of life. In your case menopause came early. We saw what was happening, worked out a Menopause Plan that was practical for your desire to avoid hormones and that worked for a pretty long time. But time passed and the changes that were happening in your body got worse."

Sofia nodded, "Yes, I'm much drier now than even a year ago."

"Yes," I said, "That's what happens, it's progressive. This year your vagina had less estrogen available than last year and so the atrophy got worse. Next year the atrophy will continue to advance. Year by year it gets drier and sex gets worse."

Sofia nodded her head indicating that she wanted me to continue.

"Women who get menopause early suffer more severe vaginal symptoms at a younger age than those for whom menopause happens later. For you, the progression of atrophy started early but in your case hormone therapy was not the right choice. For other women that would have been a good time to use low dose hormone therapy so we could delay menopause until a more average age, around fifty."

Sofia frowned a little like maybe I was putting her down but that wasn't the case at all. "Your choice was well informed and correct for you at that time, but it was limited in its benefits and that's what we're seeing now. Herbals, lubes, and natural creams all work but none of them reverse vaginal atrophy. What I see when I insert a speculum and peer around inside is pale, thin tissue that looks smooth to the touch. This is unhealthy tissue. It should be full of folds and bumps. The skin becomes inelastic. That's what we're trying to prevent. When skin loses its elasticity it becomes easy to rough up, scratch, or tear on a micro level. It might feel dry, scratchy, itchy and painful if something is inserted. So what to do? If we want to stay true to the no-hormones ethic than we need to make a new Menopause Plan," I said.

"Which would be what?" Sofia said looking at me as I looked at her.

"First, how important is sex to you?" I asked.

Sofia looked away and furrowed her brow for a long moment. "At this point in my life it's become very important actually."

"Ok, here's what I'd like to suggest then. Let's keep you hormone free as you'd like to do and let's take up where we left off talking last time."

"The Mona Lisa thing?"

"Exactly. So, what's the Mona Lisa Touch? It's a laser that treats vaginal tissue like plastic surgeons use lasers to zap wrinkled frown lines. It takes three treatments, six weeks apart. Each time we renew more and more tissue. There's no pain, downtime or anesthesia. You can have sex again five days later. No hormones needed, but I have to say we're getting the best results from the laser treatment combined with a low dose cream, but it's not necessary, just beneficial."

Sofia looked at me, "That's it?"

"Yes, your vaginal atrophy will be reversed and the new tissue will be like that of a younger woman who has yet to experience menopause."

"Why didn't we do that before?" She asked.

"You weren't having sex before. Now vaginal atrophy is a bigger issue that needs treatment. Your life changed, and we just changed your Menopause Plan. Time to treat your vaginal atrophy."

"Do I go to the hospital?" Sofia asked.

"No, it's in-office. Doesn't take very long. Between the forms, undressing, the procedure, getting dressed again it should take forty five minutes."

Sofia thought for a short time and then said, "Sign me up." She made an appointment at the reception desk in two weeks for her first Mona Lisa Touch.

CHAPTER 4

TRACEY

IN MY CASE it took nearly two years from the day I fell ill until I started to feel like myself again. I had been getting regular checkups, been meticulous with my hydration (Very important for kidney patients) and reacted like a panicked kitty at the slightest sign of returning symptoms. The fact was however I was now fine. My appetite needed another six months to re-activate but slowly my energy returned and the enjoyment of life that had drained out of me was slowly coming back.

Meanwhile my menopause had become a problem. I was one of those women who had it easy at first. No hot flashes, insomnia, erratic periods or anything like that. When my periods stopped I was relieved, because I'd always thought they were inconvenient and annoying. I was fairly young by the standards of menopause, but chose not to use any estrogen initially.

When Janet examined me at the time of my health scare she put me on the ring. It worked very well and I was satisfied with it. It was great that I was happy with it because realistically that was where the possibilities of treatment ended. At that time there was no laser rejuvenation yet, it wouldn't come down the technology pipeline until about a year later. So things at that point were going in a very satisfactory direction menopause-wise.

Fast-forward six months and now that I was paying more attention to the progression in my own body, I didn't like what I saw. Everything I'd been treating in other women over many years was now happening to me and I was about as happy about it as they had been. That is, not at all. Janet confirmed that things could be going better and we talked about alternatives. There wasn't really anything she knew of that I didn't know of at first. Then she said 'Did you hear about the trials going on at the Cleveland Clinic?' She told me about the science of laser rejuvenation and told me about the early results.

My reaction was disinterest. The results of the initial study were highly positive. The science seemed correct but for some reason I failed to feel a spark of professional interest. I said, 'If the FDA approves it I'll take a look at the data.' Or something equally nerdy. The reason for my lack of enthusiasm was that doctors can not use medications or technologies until they been proven safe and effective. They are available only for trials and research and that often spans many years. I assumed FDA approval would take five years or longer. And there I left it.

A short time later the Federal Drug Administration reviewed the results of the research, the laser and software package and declared it a safe, effective way to treat vaginal atrophy and approved it for that use.

The problem was I still wasn't interested, didn't understand why I would use it or why it would become anything better than what we had. After all it derived from a laser treatment for the removal of laugh lines. The whole idea of plastic surgery was foreign to me. Obstetrician-gynecologists use a lot of technology but the basic work we do is fairly straight forward even craftsman-like. So a device that plastic surgeons have been using didn't really seem adaptable to me.

Until I went to a seminar and began meeting doctors who had treated patients successfully and patients who had been treated. The results were sufficiently beneficial that I became professionally interested. After a short while I did the required training and certification and then I became a patient of the laser rejuvenation treatment myself.

After a very successful personal experience with the first treatment I knew this would become an important tool for doctors everywhere to use. Being one of the first in New York City was thrilling as it gave me the opportunity to advance an idea I had about menopause. That idea was that menopause needed a plan that would guide women from their early forties until their senior years toward good choices and good health. It was envisioned as a continually changing series of treatments that was individualized for every woman and changed as her body and needs changed over time.

The Menopause Plan that I was working on recognized menopause, as a decades long dynamic process that had no end date. At a certain point however in formulating The Menopause Plan I hit a dead end. There was a point at which menopause's advance outpaced medicine's ability to keep pace. For most woman there would inevitably come an age when vaginal atrophy would result in sexual dysfunction, thinning tissues and susceptibility to infections.

That changed dramatically with the Mona Lisa Touch. The Menopause Plan now had a way to help women remain sexually vibrant for as long as they wished. And if they were not sexually active there was also now a way to treat menopause so as to preserve vaginal health forestalling future illnesses from occurring. We had a treatment that made sex easier and more pleasurable and we had a way to keep sexually inactive patients healthy into their senior years.

The Menopause Plan was now complete. Doctors specializing in menopause can now effectively treat women from the onset of symptoms to the most senior of years in a continuum of care. Physicians and patients alike are no longer chasing symptoms one at a time and this is brand new. That is why this is the best age for older women there has ever been and for a physician specialist it is truly the Golden Age of Menopause.

KATHERINE

When Katherine decided to get the Mona Lisa I knew she was making a sound decision. We'd been speaking over time about the different treatments that were available for menopause. We had reviewed the information about atrophy, progression, hormones, non-hormonal therapies and so forth. Together we had forged a Menopause Plan for her to follow and as her needs changed so did the Plan.

Timmy was the driving force behind her decision to rejuvenate her vagina because his sex drive was guiding the relationship. Katherine enjoyed sex all her life and was disturbed when she couldn't consummate the physical side of things. The long time span between age 47 when she began menopause and 52 when she met Timmy proved significant in her experience of menopause.

For five years she did not have sexual intercourse at all. This coincided with the onset of skipped periods and little bit by little bit she had lost her sexual vibrancy during this time. Its absence had gone unnoticed until she wished to start having sex again. At that moment her vaginal health suddenly became an urgent matter.

Women are of course complete beings there is no separation between mind and body. If there is an affliction striking a certain body part the mind will also suffer from a mental or emotional reaction. The combined effect of being unsound in body and troubled in the mind leads to unhappiness. And that was how Katherine initially presented herself to me.

She had become unhappy because of her sexual dysfunction and she sought relief from both the physical ailments but also the emotional distress. By treating the body the mind would also be salved. This worked well for about six months. Katherine had become sexually vibrant once again enjoying sexual relations with Timmy. The localized vaginal estrogen therapy had improved her sex life to a significant extent.

Timmy's virility posed a new challenge to Katherine's Menopause Plan. She was happy to match his desire but the fact was her body could not keep up. He was too much for her in terms of frequency of sexual activity. If they had sex infrequently or if they had sex once and then stopped for a time, Katherine would've done fine on low dose hormone treatment possibly for years to come. Her vaginal tissues would've had a chance to bounce back but things being what they were, she now needed to choose either less sex or vaginal rejuvenation and she chose the latter.

"It was his idea actually," Katherine said as we finished reviewing the post procedure instructions.

"Timmy said you should get it done?"

"He's the chief beneficiary," Katherine said.

"After you," I pointed out.

"True," She said, " How long until we can have sex again?"

"Five long days. Then you can take it out for a test drive."

"Did you get this done?" Katherine asked.

"Ummm hmmm," I said nodding my head.

"And it works?" She asked.

"Ummm hmmm," I repeated and gestured that she should head toward the Mona Lisa room.

"Does it hurt?" Katherine asked.

"You'll feel a little buzzing, maybe a little scratchiness. Not very much discomfort at all. If you have any post treatment soreness it'll go away in a day or two. Most women don't have much or sometimes any."

The Mona Lisa suite is a room containing state-of-the-art technology specific to gynecology and the treatment of menopause. The array of technology consists of a medical laser identical to those used in facial rejuvenation, a handset and a computer with precise software for guiding the procedure and informing the physician of its operation and effects. There is a standard gynecological examination table with stirrups and that's about it.

Patients who choose to treat their vaginal atrophy with this method receive some instructions before they come in for their appointment. The first thing is to refrain from using any kind of lube or cream for one week before the procedure. It's best if pubic hair is well trimmed and one should abstain from sex 24 hours before. There is no pre-medication required.

When a woman arrives at the office for her treatment there are some standard things we need to do before getting underway. There is a handout with instructions and a consent form to sign. Then the doctor and patient meet to discuss any last minute questions. The doctor will review some very brief post-op instructions. No intercourse for five days, no hot tubs. If you're a little sore after the procedure you should skip working out. The rule is that you should resume routine activities as tolerated. If there aren't any other questions, then its time to move to the next step.

The patient goes to the bathroom and empties her bladder, changes below the waist and goes to the Mona Lisa suite. She positions herself on the exam table as the doctor adjusts some computer settings.

Maria our medical assistant already had the room prepared for us and was waiting patiently. I made the introductions and Maria helped Katherine onto the table and adjusted things as they needed to be. Meanwhile I took my seat on a low stool surrounded by high technology.

As I sat on the stool my gaze centered on the computer monitor that was displaying a number of parameters. I moved some knobs around to adjust power, depth, size and shape of the beam to treat Katherine's vagina properly. The laser hummed a little while it warmed up.

The software display indicated that everything was fine tuned and ready for operation. I took the hand piece from its sterilized packaging plugged it in, inspected it closely and looked around. Katherine seemed ready and Maria was standing by. I scanned every element from the lighting to my relative height on the stool, the laser apparatus and the display screen. Finally I put on a pair of safety goggles, "I'm all set. How about you?" I asked Katherine as I switched the laser from standby to ready.

"I'm good," She said.

And as gently as I could I inserted the wand shaped laser hand piece into her vagina and carefully calibrated it's depth. "Starting up," I said and then grew quiet as I put one hundred percent of my concentration on delivering precise pulses of laser energy to exactly the right spots.

A NEW COURSE OF TREATMENT

It didn't take much time until it became apparent that the Mona Lisa Touch technology was excellent both in its results and the ease of use for an experienced practitioner. The capabilities of the invention were greatly appreciated and as the months went by other doctors began to call and ask questions. We would discuss The Menopause Plan and how it could guide the extended period of treatment that menopause requires. We spoke of treatments chasing symptoms while vaginal atrophy progressed untreated and then we talked about laser rejuvenation. Like myself, skepticism abounded. There are many reasons for this including the too-good-to-be-true aspect, the newness aspect, the fact that it had not been publicized very effectively and the general aversion that doctors have to being on the cutting edge of high technology applications. Physicians, as they have often been termed are a rather conservative lot.

In the meantime the core of the problem remained for the millions of women every year entering the ages at which thoughts about menopause become relevant. Vaginal atrophy, on the scale of an entire population was continuing unchecked except with the standard treatments that are known to grow less effective over time. Technology had now clearly advanced but the knowledge of this new treatment had not disseminated widely among physicians.

The calls from other doctors kept coming in. Urologists needed to refer patients whose symptoms only a gynecologist could resolve. Cancer specialists needed their patients to avoid hormones but their patient's menopause symptoms also needed to be addressed. Internists needed consultations and referrals for the best ways to treat menopause in their women patients.

In many variations I spoke to them about herbals, lubes, creams, rings, SSRI's, non-hormonal solutions, low dose hormonal solutions, transdermal patches, safe systemic dosages, the need to individualize care and change treatments over time and finally when it proved appropriate for their patients, laser rejuvenation.

Before I became aware of it The Menopause Plan was turning from an idea in my head into a course of treatment that was practical, safe and effective.

KATHERINE

"Starting up," I said and began my work.

Katherine relaxed as much as anyone could in the stirrups. Then I began the first of her laser treatments. The computer-guided parameters were all set, the laser was charged and the hand piece was properly arranged inside her vagina. The hand piece is a wand shaped tool with various settings and calibration marks along with tiny ports for the discharge of the laser light energy. The device cools the laser light with a puff of air that accompanies each pulse. The patient feels a slight buzz, vibration or perhaps a slight stinging sensation, depending on the individual. The main effect is the pressure of the wand against skin and the puff of air, there is no pain involved in the procedure.

The doctor inserts the hand piece to the maximum depth in the vagina and begins using highly focused light to zap the tissues. Each area gets five zaps then the doctor rotates the hand-piece clock-wise, withdraws it a precise amount then rotates the hand-piece again, this time in a counter clock-wise direction, giving five more pulses.

Katherine was breathing deeply in and out doing a meditation exercise while I did her treatment. She was calm and didn't move around very much and that made it easier for me to do my work as swiftly as I could. In a short while I had gone from the deepest parts of Katherine's vagina to the opening. Every centimeter of vaginal atrophy had been zapped with exactly the right amount of light energy and within a short time new tissues would grow. They'll be more moist, elastic and soft and the improvements will continue for six months. Within weeks her vagina will be stronger, healthier and have regained the bumps and folds indicative of healthy vaginal tissue.

The final pulse of laser light was applied and I straightened my back and switched the laser off, Maria took the hand piece from me without being asked and I said, "We're done."

"That's it?" Katherine replied as she took her feet from the stirrups.

"You are good to go," I said shutting off the computer. Katherine went off to get dressed, Maria began the sterilization procedure and I retreated to my office to make notes, say goodbye to Katherine when she emerged from the dressing room, and got ready to see the next patient who would be delivering her third child in May.

Katherine didn't call me. I didn't hear a word from her after the procedure and for doctors silence is the same as thunderous applause is to an actor. Silence means 'I don't have any medical issues and everything is fine, therefore I don't need to think about the doctor call them or make an appointment.' Doctors usually hear immediately when an issue has arisen and Katherine's silence meant she had forgotten about me. Just as it should be.

Skepticism generally lasts until evidence dissolves it. In the face of hard facts it becomes difficult to favor one's mental formations over truthful things. And so over time my own skepticism changed. I had gone from being disinterested in laser rejuvenation, to being a willing listener to its benefits to being a woman treated by it.

In other words, my skepticism had resolved enough that I was treated myself before I treated any of my patients. I had reviewed the science behind it extensively. My experience of menopause made me a perfect candidate, I was the right age and my symptoms could be fixed with this remedy. Yet it took a leap of faith to be among the first women who were treated with it.

And that was where the skepticism ended. My knowledge was no longer based on reading technical literature and reviewing studies or listening to other doctors and hearing testimonials. My education in laser rejuvenation was now complete. I knew the science, had trained in the technical aspects, read the studies and then completed the last phase with a personal tryout.

This was vitally important to me as I would never recommend a treatment, medication or procedure I would not prescribe for myself, my mother, my family or my friends. Doing no harm is a medical credo but it goes deeper, it is also a personal vow that physicians take. If the Mona Lisa Touch produced anything other than the tangible benefits it promised, it would not be useful for either myself or other gynecologists.

The results speak for themselves. From a patient's point of view, the procedure is fast, painless and requires no anesthesia or downtime. The vast majority of women who have been treated see marked improvement in their vagina's health within a short period. This continues to improve for up to six months. After the second and third treatments there is a significant amount of new, moist, strong, elastic vaginal tissue where little or none existed before. A number of women will see smaller improvements from the first treatment but by the time they have completed the full course their vaginas will also share similar results to the early good responders.

From a doctor's perspective, menopause can now be treated from beginning to end and this is an entirely new thing in gynecology, it didn't exist before the year 2015. As I contemplated the results of the laser rejuvenation therapy it struck me that eventually almost every woman could benefit from this method of treatment.

The Mona Lisa Touch may be the first laser treatment approved for vaginal atrophy but there will surely be others in the years to come and they will all represent a tremendous leap forward in women's health.

The next time I saw Katherine was for her second and eventually her third treatment. These were scheduled six weeks apart and she responded very well to each treatment. She reported that she didn't experience any discomfort and each time yielded marked improvement. Examination after examination proved the same thing, Katherine's vaginal tissues were rejuvenating themselves. Healthy cells were now taking over where atrophic cells once were.

Layer by layer the effects were deepening creating soft, moist tissue that had a high degree of elasticity, abundant bumps and folds. Her vagina had changed from that commonly found in older women to the kind of vagina commonly found in younger women. It had become the type of vaginal tissue that allows for pleasurable sex, easier orgasmic potential and greater resistance to infection. In short, Katherine now had a healthy vagina because her atrophy had been reversed.

NADIA

Nadia was from Czechoslovakia and she was notable for her aristocratic bearing, exquisite fashion sense and a sparkling wit that matched her diamonds. Remarkable as those characteristics were she was also seventy-nine years old and sexually active. Her newest boyfriend was twenty years younger than her and came from an old line Philadelphia family. They were living together in her apartment on Fifth Avenue and she made an appointment one day to see me.

"Sweetie!" She purred as she gave me the slightest of embraces and a pair of air kisses.

"Hello Nadia. How's Binky?" I asked.

"Fine, he's in the Cayman Islands setting up a shell company and he's going to be gone for two weeks so I thought I'd give him a surprise and you're it."

"Me?"

"Yes, my darling you." Nadia took a glossy women's magazine from her oversized Gucci handbag and showed me the section she'd earmarked. It was the first article I'd ever seen in the public press about laser rejuvenation and I stared at it for a few seconds before looking up.

"Do me," She said, "Today possible?"

I looked at her and had to smile. She was as old as my Grandmother was when I was just starting medical school and she had a boyfriend, researched a remedy for herself and wanted to surprise Binky with a rejuvenated vagina when he returned from his business trip.

Nadia, I suddenly realized was an icon for a new kind of older woman. Someone I don't believe my Grandmother would have recognized, nor considered as a role model for herself. Nadia was the living embodiment of a woman who had indeed both aged gracefully and retained her sexual vibrancy right up to her eighth decade. I was wondering if she and I would be having a similar discussion near her hundredth birthday.

I looked up from Nadia's chart and asked, "Have you used any creams or lubricants for the past week?"

"No darling, I know it's verboten."

I nodded and signaled that I'd be right back. I went to the receptionist's desk, looked at the schedule, checked for texts and messages, called the Chief Resident to make sure everything at the hospital was good and my presence was not needed. I returned to my office and said, "Yes we can fit you in. Maria will help you fill out some forms, you'll need to empty your bladder, disrobe below the waist, go to the Mona Lisa suite and then we'll be all ready."

Nadia smiled broadly and asked me sotto voce as we passed close by in the doorway, "My love, have you had this done yet to yourself?"

"Ummm hmmmm," I replied.

"On the scale of good things from one to ten with ten being the best of good things how would you rate it?"

"Ummmm, ten," I replied, "Still want to do this?"

"Oh yes," Nadia said, "Binky will be so surprised."

I didn't say it out loud because my mind was already leaping forward to the things I needed to do to get ready. But what I was thinking was, 'You and him both.'

GWYNETH

The last patient I saw that week came in late on a Friday. It had been a long week with a Caesarean section, many office visits, lab results and a number of procedures. I was looking forward to the weekend. Gwyneth was ushered into my office by the ever-smiling Maria and she took a seat opposite me in the office. She was forty-eight years old and we talked idly for a moment or two. She was a music teacher at a high school in the Village and she grew up in Florida where I have family. After a short while I asked the Interval Medical History questions and when we got to the sex part, she got a quizzical look on her face.

"Doctor Fein," She said, "Every time me and my boyfriend have sex I get a yeast infection. It hurts it goes away it comes back. I mean every time."

"Why don't we go and have a look and see what's going on?" I said, and Gwyneth and I made our way to the exam room. I conducted a routine examination, took a sample from her cervix for a Pap and said that she should get dressed and afterward meet me back in my office.

She did that and when she was seated before me, I began to speak with her as I speak with many of my women patients these days. I said to Gwyneth, "The time has come for us to talk about a Menopause Plan because the symptoms you were describing arise from the fact that your menopause has begun and the discomfort you feel when having sex is due to vaginal atrophy, not a yeast infection."

Gwyneth's mouth dropped open slightly at the sound of these words and her head tilted a little to one side. I continued on, "We can treat this but what I really want to talk to you about is what the road ahead offers and what you and I can do together to make it as smooth and easy as possible." She straightened up slightly in her chair and looked at me, "All right, I'm listening," She said.

CONCLUSION

DOCTOR'S BEST ADVICE

THE BEST ADVICE a doctor can give to women undergoing menopause is clear and simple. With proper treatment menopause can be a gentle process that interweaves itself with the rest of a woman's natural life. Find a physician menopause specialist who can guide and coach you through this period providing The Menopause Plan that is best for you. Every woman experiences menopause differently and the most beneficial Plan is an individualized one that changes over time as the effects of menopause itself, changes over time.

Best wishes for good health. Dr. Tracey Fein, M.D.

TheMenopausePlan.com

Made in the USA
Charleston, SC
15 February 2017